Dr. Newbold's
TYPE A/TYPE B
WEIGHT LOSS BOOK

Dr. Newbold's

TYPE A / TYPE B

WEIGHT
LOSS BOOK

H. L. Newbold, M.D.

KEATS PUBLISHING, INC.
NEW CANAAN, CONNECTICUT

Dr. Newbold's Type A/Type B Weight Loss Book is not intended
as medical advice. Its intent is solely informational
and educational. Please consult a health professional
should the need for one be indicated.

Library of Congress Cataloging-in-Publication Data

Newbold, H. L. (Herbert Leon)
[Type A/type B weight loss book.]
Dr. Newbold's Type A/type B weight loss book : about people
who love foods and the foods that hate them / by H.L. Newbold ;
preface by Linus Pauling.
p.   cm.
Includes bibliographical references and index.
ISBN 0-87983-550-8 : $10.95
1. Reducing diets.   2. Animal food—Fat content.   3. Food habits.
I. Title.   II. Title: Doctor Newbold's type A/type B weight loss book.
RM222.2.N483   1991
613.2'5—dc20   91–22116
CIP

Printed in the United States of America

Published by Keats Publishing, Inc.
27 Pine Street (P. O. Box 876)
New Canaan, Connecticut 06840-0876

For
The Next Generation:

Martha Saunders
Ruth Saunders

Geoffrey Corley
Peter Corley

Acknowledgments

The author is grateful to
Pat Connolly and William Baker
for reading the manuscript of this book
and offering valuable suggestions.

Contents

Foreword

We need to concentrate on the health of the appestat mechanism instead of calorie counting and the sheer exercise of willpower. Fight obesity without nature's help—without an adequate appestat mechanism—is like traveling up a swift-flowing river in a rowboat.

Roger Williams, Ph.D.
Professor Emeritus of Biochemistry
University of Texas at Austin
Formerly president of the
American Chemical Society

Author's Note

Please Read This First

Your next door neighbor can give you all sorts of medical and nutritional advice without taking a history, doing a physical examination, or ordering laboratory tests. If the advice works, fine. If not . . . well, it just didn't work out.

A physician, however, is expected to take the full responsibility for whatever medical advice he gives.

For this reason, when writing a book on a medical subject, I must give advice that applies generally. I cannot directly give any one personal medical advice without first taking a medical history, doing a physical examination, and ordering laboratory tests.

Since it is not possible for me to carry out these procedures before allowing you to read this book, I must *insist* that you check with your physician before taking any of the advice given in this book. Your physician knows you and should be able to judge whether or not the medical advice contained between these covers is appropriate for you. If you undertake any treatment plan given in this book—or in any other book—your physician should work with you and follow your progress.

Your physician, the doctor who examines you, must take the responsibility for your health and anything you do to improve it.

To preserve their privacy, the names and identifying facts about patients mentioned in this book have been changed.

Those of you who read the complete book—and I hope all of you will—might notice that a few points are repeated several times. I have purposefully made the repetitions because they deal with crucial points that a pick-and-chose reader might miss.

H. L. Newbold, M.D.
New York, New York

Preface

Dr. H. L. Newbold has called on his extensive experience and wide knowledge to write an interesting and valuable book on weight reduction.

This book is unusual because of his recommendation of a diet high in animal fat to reduce cholesterol and help control overweight.

I recommend it to persons with a weight problem because of its value, and to other readers because the many facts that he presents are interesting.

I strongly recommend this book.

Linus Pauling, Ph.D.
Nobel Laureate
Linus Pauling Institute of Science and Medicine

Introduction

This book was written by a nutritionist with an interest in obesity, something few specialists have been able to do anything about. Certainly there are as many diets and theories of nutrition as there are specialists—each has his own favored approach, some of which are suspicious and possibly harmful. But this author has come up with something new, something new based on an old idea: that the human organism began to differentiate from related anthropoids well over a million years ago and that not only did gross morphology (the shape and form of our bodies) evolve but that our endocrine and digestive systems adapted to the environments of early humans. Dr. Newbold's theory (oversimplified and taken out of context) is that we should avoid "new" foods such as the grains that came in in the Neolithic Age and stick to those foods we are most adapted to: meats and, of all things, animal fat. He believes that the obese are intolerant of the newer foods. He makes a good case for his theory.

While I am not obese, I enjoyed this book. It has an easy and natural style and I learned a few things to boot. I don't ordinarily go in for puns, but there is plenty to chew on here for those who need to lose weight and who have given up on the run-of-the-mill cures.

The authorities cited and those listed in the bibliography are for the most part highly respected, and there are certainly enough of them to suit the most demanding readers. It was good to see a familiar name, that of Dr. Roger Williams, one of the greats in the nutrition field and a courageous innovator who was not afraid to strike out on his own. Innovation is never easy. It can be lonely. When one is both introducing and using new paradigms, one's work is bound to be controversial, which I'm sure will be nothing new for Dr. Newbold.

One last note: While Newbold may be didactic, this book gives the impression that he can use his head and that he does not take his patients' welfare lightly.

Edward T. Hall, Ph.D.
Professor Emeritus (Anthropology)
Northwestern University

Dr. Newbold's
TYPE A/TYPE B
WEIGHT LOSS BOOK

1

Do You Have a *Type-A* or a *Type-B* Weight Problem?

It's the person you like best and the food you like best that give you the most trouble.

—H. L. NEWBOLD

Type-A (The Spree Eater)

Have you ever eaten a piece of cake or a few scoops of ice cream and found yourself more hungry instead of less hungry? After eating the goodie, did you suddenly turn so ravenously hungry you were ready to gobble down a Golden Gate Bridge made of cake—and have a chocolate ice cream Twin Towers for dessert?

If so, you're a spree eater. If you're overweight, you have a *Type-A* weight problem. Here's what happens: because of a sensitivity problem, the food that made you hungry knocked out the appestat center in your brain, the center that tells us when we're hungry and when we've had enough to eat. Without a properly working appestat, we're like machines without a governor. We become insatiable eating machines.

Ounces and pounds put on during eating sprees stay with us and we become overweight.

You'll be happy to learn that you can solve your hunger problem, your appestat problem, and regain and forever keep the slender figure of a gold medal gymnast.

1

Type-B (The Addictive Eater)

Does a strong urge to eat a *particular* food—cookies, for example—sometimes strike you? You want *that food* and *no other*. Is your desire for cookies so compelling that you'd fight the Iraqi Army across the desert sands of Saudi Arabia to get your hands on a box of the delicious sugar-coated treat? Do you get weak and shaky, find you can't concentrate, feel you'll explode in anger or fall apart and end up in ten thousand pieces if you don't soon eat your favorite treat?

If so, you're an addictive eater. If you're overweight, you have a *Type-B* weight problem. Forces that you don't understand are at work inside you. They drive you to repeatedly eat a fattening food and make you put on unwanted pounds.

Follow the directions in this book and you will lose your addiction to foods and become addicted to life.

Many doubly unlucky people—as I did—have a mixed *Type-A* and *Type-B* weight problem. They too can lose two to three pounds a week and stay slender forever.

I Know Because I was Fat and Now I'm Not

I know firsthand about the problem of being overweight, and I know firsthand about the laws of nature that we must follow to lose weight. Twenty years ago, I was overweight. I had always been slender until I began interning at the University of Chicago. Night and day we labored, 95 hours a week. They gave us $104 to buy uniforms. That was all the money they paid us for the year. However, we had "free" laundry, "free" room, and "free" food.

With so little pleasure, so much work, and so little money, guess what we did for fun? We ate. We stood in the cafeteria line to choose a regular meal, then we went back not once but several times for more jelly sweet rolls, more cherry tarts, more apple pie à la mode. The more we ate, the more we were being paid, or so it seemed.

Some of us became addicted to certain carbohydrates, to foods that contained sugar, grains, or milk.

As doctors we should have known better than to put on extra weight, but we were young and our thoughts were elsewhere. We told ourselves that other people got fat. We got "chubby." At six-foot-one I became not just chubby, but a fat 232 pounds.

How I Was Motivated To Lose Weight

By the time I arrived at middle age, heart attacks had dropped several of my friends. A great truism began descending upon me: I too might not be immortal. Still, not motivated strongly enough, I did nothing to lose weight.

Then modern man's most dreaded pain struck me in the chest, a sharp, expanding pain I had never felt before. I turned weak and sweaty. The big "H," a heart attack.

I spent the next four weeks at the wrong end of the medical establishment: as a patient in the hospital. Nurses smiled, doctors thumped and I wondered whether I would make it through the night.

When I returned home I was determined both to lose weight and to lower my high cholesterol. I would completely turn my life around and survive.

I followed conventional medical wisdom: To lose weight, I reduced the amount of calories I ate. To lower my cholesterol, I left off red meats and saturated fats.

On the second day of my new diet I felt irritable, restless, and dissatisfied. I daydreamed about the mounds of ice cream I had eaten as an intern. Nevertheless, I clung to my plan.

At four in the morning of the third day of my new diet, a vague discomfort awakened me. It was not a pain like I had known earlier, but, as before, I felt water-weak and sweaty. A sense of doom engulfed me. The siren screamed again as the ambulance carried me back to the hospital for what I thought was a second heart attack.

Tests were negative. Sometimes, however, it takes a day or two for tests to show damage. They would repeat the tests the next day.

That night in the hospital a sedative settled me down for sleep. At 4:45 a.m., however, I awakened tense and sweaty. Although I had no pain, again I had a strong feeling that disaster was about to descend on me.

A student nurse checked my blood pressure.

"Could I have another sleeping pill?"

"I'll ask the charge nurse as soon as she gets back. Meanwhile, I'll bring you a glass of orange juice."

I shook my head. "It will make me put on weight."

"It might help you relax and go back to sleep. You can worry about your weight later. You need a good night's sleep."

"Maybe you're right."

She returned with a tall glass of delicious, sugar-laden orange juice.

She was right. Before the senior nurse returned, my tense muscles began melting and I slid into the best sleep of the night.

That afternoon, a new set of tests reports came back normal and I returned home.

Two days after returning home the whole show repeated itself: the sweating, the anxiety, the feeling of doom. Sirens pushed cars aside as an ambulance sped me back to the hospital. Again the tests were negative.

Clearly, my doctor and the consultants he called to examine me did not know what was wrong. Finally, my doctor suggested, "Maybe you're having anxiety attacks. I'd like to try you on a tranquilizer."

I did not know what was causing my symptoms, but I did know that I was not suffering from anxiety attacks.

Again when I awakened at four in the morning with tension, sweating, and the feeling that I was about to die, the nurse gave me a sugar-laden glass of orange juice. As before, I relaxed and went back to sleep.

After I returned home, at dawn the second day the heavy scene repeated: the cold sweats, the weakness, the doom. When absolutely forced to, we use our heads. While the biochemical storm whirled through me, I sat in bed and tried to think. I considered wild diagnoses, all the way from Adams-Stokes disease to Ziehen-Oppenheim disease.

Addiction And Withdrawal

I now know that I was struggling with a *Type-B* weight problem, a food addiction. That discovery, however, was a painful process. Here's how I began learning about it. As I sat in bed thinking, a memory began coming to me from the back roads of my mind. Somewhere I had read about addictions to carbohydrate foods such as sugar, wheat and milk. Perhaps addiction to carbohydrates followed the same rules as an addiction to narcotics, like morphine or heroin.

Angry, restless, depressed, nauseated, sweating: you've seen movies that show how people suffer when they withdraw from narcotics. Withdrawal symptoms can include almost any symptom known to man. The narcotic addict must have his narcotic, his "fix" at regular intervals to avoid withdrawal symptoms. *To avoid withdrawal symptoms, the narcotic addict must not only have his fix, but he must have it in adequate amounts.*

While suffering withdrawal symptoms, *if the drug addict gets his fix in a large enough amount,* immediately he loses all unpleasant symptoms. He feels at peace with himself and the world—until his withdrawal symptoms return and he needs another fix to feel right again.

Food Addictions

Like the heroin addict, I reasoned, perhaps the person addicted to certain carbohydrates must eat *adequate amounts* of his addictive food at regular intervals to avoid withdrawal symptoms. To lose weight I had cut down on the *amount* of carbohydrate I ate. If I had an addiction to grains, sugar, or milk and failed to eat *adequate amounts* of grains, sugar, or milk at frequent intervals, I might suffer withdrawal symptoms.

I remembered the nurse who fed me the sugar-spiked orange juice in the hospital. Perhaps she had given me the fix I needed. Maybe that was why my symptoms disappeared. In any case, I knew how to test and learn whether my mysterious attacks were caused by withdrawal from certain carbohydrates.

The Test

While I lay in bed still sweating and feeling as if I were balanced insecurely on the edge of the world, I asked for a heaping dish of apple pie à la mode. The treat would give me milk, sugar and wheat, an almost perfect carbohydrate fix.

Before I finished eating the gooey mess of delicious wickedness, all of my symptoms faded, including the frightening sense of doom. I stopped sweating. I smiled. All was right with the world. At last I had the correct diagnosis: *I was addicted to carbohydrates. When I had cut down on the amount of carbohydrates I ate to lose weight, it brought on withdrawal symptoms.*

Doctors Don't Know

I questioned my internist. As I suspected, he knew nothing about addictive foods and withdrawal reactions. He found the subject boring.

"Take a Valium and forget about food addictions," he advised.

I began telephoning doctors around the country to pick their minds. An old friend in Chicago remembered something about food addictions and withdrawal reactions. He thought he had read about it in a newspaper.

"As I recall," he told me, *"people get addicted to certain carbohydrates. They don't become addicted to fresh meats. I don't remember the details."*

New Approach

To cure my addiction, this time I would try totally removing carbohydrates such as grains, milk products and table sugar from my diet. I would eat a fish-fowl-meat-raw vegetable-raw fruit diet. If my reasoning was correct, like an addict withdrawing from heroin, I would feel ill for three or four days and then be finished with withdrawal symptoms— as well as my addiction.

On the second day of my new diet, sweat beaded my forehead. Restlessness, irritability and a sensation of approaching doom struck me. I yearned for mounds of wonderfully soft and slurpy ice cream. Instead of rushing for the delicious treat, I simply lay around the house and hung on.

If my theory was correct, these were withdrawal symptoms. They would end after three or four days. On the third day the symptoms began fading. On the fourth day, the weakness and gloom lifted. I felt as if I had crossed over the high mountain passes into peaceful Shangri La.

There was no question about what had happened: I had been withdrawing from the carbohydrates to which I was addicted. Now I had beaten the withdrawal awfuls. I had more energy. And I was no longer hungry.

I reasoned that I had become overweight because I had been eating certain carbohydrates (carbohydrates to which I was addicted) at *frequent intervals* and in *large amounts to avoid withdrawal symptoms.*

By leaving most carbohydrates out of my diet, I had conquered what I later came to call a *Type-B* weight problem, addictive eating. To my surprise, my excess weight began disappearing at the rate of two or three pounds a week.

Why Most People With Type-B Weight Problems Fail To Lose Weight

People with *Type-B* weight problems have withdrawal symptoms when they go on calorie-cutting diets. They feel terrible. Neither the patients nor their physicians know that they are experiencing withdrawal symptoms.

Neither the patients nor their physicians know that their symptoms will disappear within three or four days. (In rare cases, withdrawal symptoms may last for a week. However, on the other hand, many people have withdrawal symptoms much milder than mine. They may feel irritable and get in arguments with their associates and mates, or find it impossible to concentrate.)

To keep from worrying about my nutritional needs, I placed myself on a generous intake of vitamins, minerals and adequate amounts of unsaturated fats.

My New Dilemma: Cholesterol

Clearly, I had broken my addiction to carbohydrates, but if I ate red meats wouldn't my already high cholesterol level shoot through the roof?

If a doctor stops at an automobile accident and finds a patient with a broken nose and a cut artery in the leg pumping blood, what does he do? He treats the most threatening injury first. He stops the bleeding, then he turns his attention to the broken nose.

The withdrawal reactions associated with the low-carbohydrate diet had been disabling me. For that reason I had to eat the fish-fowl-meat-raw vegetable-raw fruit diet. Even if such a diet made my cholesterol climb, I had to solve my most pressing problem first. Later, I would try to lower my cholesterol.

Statistics said that within the five years following a heart attack, half of the patients were carried out the exit door. I had little to lose. I felt free to experiment with my body.

When I visited my internist's office for a checkup, he complimented me on my appearance and my weight loss. My weight had fallen to 221.

I told him I was taking vitamins and eating a fish-fowl-meat-raw vegetable-raw fruit diet. "I feel best on fatty rib steaks."

"Eating fatty steaks after having a heart attack!"

"Maybe I'm killing myself," I said, "but I feel great and my weight's falling."

"What about your cholesterol?"

"Who knows?"

"Let's check it."

"Not yet. I have a hunch that I'm about to make a discovery. We don't know much about the effects of foods on body chemistry. I'm groping my way."

I had a gut feeling that I was doing the right thing. Experience had taught me to wait a long time before going against my gut feelings. Our brains might not be the smartest part of our body.

I felt healthy and my weight kept falling two to three pounds a week. No matter what my cholesterol level might be, I was not going to change my diet. Curiosity, however, finally sent me to a lab for another cholesterol test.

The lab reported my cholesterol was under 200! My cholesterol had been 312 when I had my coronary. They must have confused my blood sample with someone else's. Maybe they used outdated chemicals or a broken machine. I went to another lab: cholesterol under 200. Still not satisfied, I visited the hospital lab where they had performed my first cholesterol tests: 192.

I had to believe it. Now suddenly I felt more secure and 20 years younger in spirit as well as in body. I had made a great discovery: I could eat fatty steaks and lower my cholesterol *if* I followed a fish-fowl-meat-raw vegetable-raw fruit diet; *if* I left all grains, table sugar, milk and milk products out of my diet; and *if* I took vitamins and other nutritional supplements.

In spite of having eaten a high red meat, high animal fat diet for 20 years my last cholesterol reading was 132.

To my surprise, entirely without any effort—as if by magic, my weight kept falling at the rate of two to three pounds a week. My weight is now 176. Effortlessly, for 20 years I've kept my weight normal.

Eat Red Meat and Animal Fat—and Lower Cholesterol?

I told the cardiologist that I had discovered a new way to lower cholesterol: by eating fatty steaks. His eyes blanked out and his mind cut off. This was beyond his understanding.

I told other doctors how I ate fatty meats and lowered my cholesterol, and lost weight. They couldn't understand it either.

Aside from losing my own excess weight, back in 1969 I had little interest in weight problems. Lowering my weight and my cholesterol probably saved my life. That was good enough for me. Why struggle against the medical establishment to point out its errors?

Now, 20 years later, I'm more interested in weight reduction and teaching physicians about my new way to lower weight and lower cholesterol. I've had scientific articles published about my cholesterol research in respected, mainstream, peer-reviewed, Medical-Index listed medical journals such as the *International Journal for Vitamin and Nutrition Research* and the *Southern Medical Journal*. I reported on well-controlled cases. I've had hundreds of other patients, however, who ate a high animal fat diet and lowered their cholesterol levels or maintained their already low cholesterol levels. I have one patient who, with the exception of a baked potato once a month at the time of her menstrual period, could eat only beef rib steaks. When she first visited me 10 years ago, her cholesterol level was 180. It's still 180.

I later discovered that people who are *not* overweight can also lower their cholesterol levels by following a diet of fresh fish-fowl-meat-raw vegetable-raw fruit diet.

Most physicians still shake their heads when I talk about my discovery. They don't understand my findings. They fail to understand because:

1. They've never treated and observed a patient who ate no grains, no milk or milk products, and no table sugar.

2. They are not well enough informed about evolution and anthropology (the study of early man, who passed not only his body form but

his biochemistry along to us) to understand the theory I've developed to explain my discovery.

The Medical Establishment Rejects New Discoveries

The medical world has never been receptive to highly original discoveries that disrupt the status quo, that turn the power structure upside down.

When Harvey discovered that blood circulates, his fellow physicians rejected his findings. It took 199 years before the medical world accepted them.

During the middle of the last century, Ignaz Semmelweis worked at the general hospital in Vienna. As a young doctor he challenged authority and conventional wisdom when he proved that doctors who went from performing autopsies to delivering babies without washing their hands were infecting mothers and giving them deadly childbed fever.

As a reward for his great discovery, he was ridiculed and dismissed from his post. He wandered the streets of Vienna urging women not to risk their lives by going to the hospital to have their babies. Eventually, Semmelweis went insane. He returned to his native country of Hungary and suicided.

A generation later Pasteur confirmed that bacteria caused infections. The medical profession nodded its head and said, "Oh, yes, Semmelweis was right." The profession then adopted Semmelweis as one of its honored saints.

The Bellevue Hospital Experiment

Years after I made my discovery, I read about an all-meat diet conducted as a research project in 1928 at Bellevue Hospital under the direction of famed Eugene F. Du Bois, M.D., Professor of Physiology, Cornell University Medical School. The experiment was carried out on Vilhjalmur Stefansson, an anthropologist. Twenty percent of Stefansson's calories came from protein and 80 percent from animal fat. C. W. Liels, M. D., assembled a group of doctors to examine Stefansson to learn whether the meat diet had harmed him. On July 3, 1926 the *Journal of* the *American Medical Association* published the result of the examination. The controlled study revealed that while eating nothing but meat and animal fat for 12 months, Stefansson's cholesterol fell 51 mg!

If you wish, you can follow my diet without eating any red meat. Fowl such as chicken and geese, or fish can be eaten in place of the red meat.

Later in the book I'll tell you how to manage the impurities in meat and how to avoid the cancer threats associated with meat and animal fat.

Why Meat Fats?

Fats (such as those found in fowl, fish and red meats), unlike carbohydrates such as spaghetti and ice cream, do not cause addictions. Thus we are not driven to eat fats at close intervals and in large amounts to avoid withdrawal symptoms. We automatically limit calories. We do not develop *Type-B* (addictive) overweight problems from fats.

In a later chapter I will explain why fats do not cause *Type-A* (spree eating) weight problems either. (I later learned that I suffered from a *Type-A* as well as *Type-B* weight problem.)

Fats have more than twice as many calories as carbohydrates, foods such as sugar, wheat, potatoes, and fruits. Conventional wisdom says that reducing fats in the diet is essential for people who want to lose weight.

That *sounds* logical, doesn't it? *But it's not true.*

In real life, eating fats helps you lose weight—*but only if you make a deep cut in the carbohydrates you eat. Fats have more calories, but fats satisfy your hunger four or five times as much as carbohydrates.* That's one of several reasons why eating fats help people lose weight.

Once you understand the principles, weight loss is simple. In a chapter near the end of the book, I've hidden a tip on losing weight that I've never told anyone until now.

2

Patients Teach Me More About How to Lose Weight

> *If we all worked on the assumption that what is accepted as true is true, there would be little hope of advance.*
> —ORVILLE WRIGHT

MARY LOU MASTERSON

Soon after working out my diet and returning to my practice, a desperate woman brought her 23-year-old daughter to see me. Mary Lou's pale skin had a dough-like quality. Her slack face and body, coupled with her hooded eyelids made her look as if she would fall asleep at any moment. And she was overweight. Not just chubby, but overflowing-the-chair fat.

The mother gave me the history. Mary Lou had been bottle-fed as an infant. From the first, she had suffered from colic, irritability, insomnia, intermittent diarrhea and moodiness, suggesting that milk was incompatible with her chemistry.

During her teens Mary Lou's personality began moving back and forth between moody periods when she sat and stared at nothing, and periods when she had bursts of uncontrolled rage. Several times a year her family had to confine her to a psychiatric hospital where she would, after a week, become wide awake, pleasant and bright. Incidentally, she always lost weight while in the hospital.

Because of my growing interest in nutrition, I had devoured many

12

books and articles on the subject. Some of them dealt with cerebral allergies, patients whose brain chemistry was disrupted by food incompatibilities.

I asked the mother about the patient's diet. Milk was the only food that truly interested Mary Lou, gallons of glorious milk. She drank milk many times every day, up to four gallons of milk a day. Clearly, she was addicted to milk.

"How much milk would you drink when you were in the hospital?" I asked.

She shrugged her shoulders. "Just a little bit."

At home she drank massive amounts of milk and became emotionally ill. In the hospital she had very little milk and lost her symptoms.

Possible conclusion: A large amount of milk was incompatible with her chemistry and gave her cerebral symptoms. Such reactions to foods have often been documented in the medical literature.

Mary Lou had been treated by more than half a dozen psychiatrists. Using psychotherapy and medication, none of them had been able to give her any permanent help. Contrary to what most people know, the sugars in milk make it a high-carbohydrate food. Why not take Mary Lou off milk and observe what happened? What did she have to lose?

When the young woman heard that I wanted her to stop drinking milk, she wanted nothing more to do with me. She pushed up from the chair and waddled toward the door.

The mother rushed over to her, turned her around and waddled her back.

"Milk might be toxic for you and interfere with your brain chemistry," I explained.

The mother nodded as if she understood and agreed. From the look on her face, however, I suspected that she thought I was talking nonsense. But this was the only new approach she had heard and she was willing to give it a try.

I explained that because Mary Lou was addicted to milk, she would have marked withdrawal symptoms when she stopped drinking it.

Two days later I got a call from the mother. In a cold tone, she cancelled the next appointment. After leaving off milk, Mary Lou had been worse than ever. She had to take Mary Lou back to the hospital.

"Do you remember that I told you she would be sick for a few days? She probably had withdrawal symptoms. It takes at least four days for a food to leave the body. You shouldn't expect Mary Lou to improve right away. Why don't you try to keep her off the milk when she comes home from the hospital?"

"Maybe," the mother said. Her voice held no determination.

That, I thought, was the last I would ever hear of Mary Lou. Too bad, I might have changed her life.

Mary Lou Revisited

Four months later Mary Lou's mother telephoned again. "You've got to do something for Mary Lou."

"I can't do anything. *You* have to do something."

Mary Lou had gotten worse. She was now in the hospital for the third time since seeing me. "And she's coming home tomorrow."

"Don't let her have any milk."

Two days later the mother called to tell me that she had locked a chain around the refrigerator, but Mary Lou pried off the handle, slipped the chain down and polished off five quarts of milk.

"Look," I advised, "put one chain around the refrigerator front to back, and one side to side. Lock the ends of the chain and then lock the chains together where they cross each other."

After hanging up, I wondered what my ex-professor of psychiatry would say if he had overheard the conversation. Probably he'd say, "Newbold always did have to try different approaches. He'll either end up in jail or win a Nobel Prize."

You guessed right. Things did not go smoothly. We had our struggles, but after a no-milk week Mary Lou looked and felt like a different person. Her skin turned pink, her eyes cleared, she took a bath and for the first time began helping her mother with the household chores.

She went off her diet several times and even had one trip back to the hospital, but she finally learned that milk was poison for her.

By eating a fish-fowl-meat-limited vegetable diet, *within eight months, Mary Lou lost nearly a hundred pounds.* Because at the time I was concerned primarily with her emotional state and had little interest in weight reduction per se, I didn't think much about her weight loss. Now I realize that she suffered from what I have come to call a *Type-B* (addictive) weight problem.

Postscript

About three years later, I got a note from Mary Lou bringing me up to date and asking me to fill out a reference form. She had left home and now lived in Louisville.

A couple of years later she sent me a wedding picture. Her eyes were bright and full of life. She was slender and almost pretty. Later she sent me a photograph of her baby. "I'm nursing her," she said. "I'm not going to give her any cow's milk."

Another year flashed by. This time she enclosed a note, but no photograph. The little one was doing fine. Her husband had left her. "Well, that's how it goes, I guess," her note said in closing.

I crossed my fingers and hoped she wouldn't fall apart.

Then I heard from Mary Lou again. During her divorce she had started drinking milk. It made her gain weight and feel strange. She stopped drinking it. She enclosed a picture of her new husband, the owner of a cafe in Cincinnati. "He's much better than my first husband. I'm expecting again. I guess I'm what anybody would call happy."

That's the last I ever heard from Mary Lou. She faded into the midlands. She had her own life. The past was past.

Gradually I began to understand that food incompatibilities revealed themselves in many different forms. They gave one person mental and emotional symptoms. The next person developed high blood pressure, headaches, arthritis, or insomnia, high cholesterol—and/or weight problems.

It wasn't until years later that I fully realized that I had stumbled onto the key to weight loss.

MRS. RINALDI

Mrs. Rinaldi (we'll call her here), was a nice little roly-poly, menopausal-age Park Avenue woman who consulted me. For 30 years headaches had ruined her life.

"I don't know why I'm bothering you about my headaches," she told me during her first visit. "Last night my husband and I sat down and added up the number of doctors I've consulted. We counted 51, but I'm sure we missed a few. I know I'm wasting my money, but unless I keep trying, I'll suffer from headaches for the rest of my life."

I've done every imaginable kind of test for food incompatibilities, all the way from skin tests to blood tests. None is wholly satisfactory. I now have patients eat one food at a time in a controlled manner and observe the effect.

A test meal of wheat made Mrs. Rinaldi retreat into her darkened bedroom with an ice pack on her forehead and enough medication to slide her into La-La Land. We had the answer to preventing her headaches.

At first Mrs. Rinaldi and I were both so pleased about curing her headaches that we didn't notice her balloon-like hips and thighs were slimming down.

"My stomach seems to have shrunk," she told me. "I'm completely satisfied with half as much food."

In addition to her headaches, we learned that she suffered from what I call a *Type-B* weight problem, addictive eating. She had a compulsion to eat wheat-containing foods such as bread, pasta and cake.

After removing all traces of wheat from her diet, for two months Mrs. Rinaldi had no headaches. Then she decided to perform a test on her own. On New Year's Eve she and her husband went to an elegant party at the Plaza where she drank a bit too much champagne.

She giddily told her husband near midnight, "I don't believe it really was wheat that gave me headaches. I think they were psychosomatic."

Her husband begged her not to eat anything with wheat in it. He urged her to go home, but she was past reasoning. She had another glass of champagne.

Then she told him she was leaving to powder her nose. On her way to the washroom, she sneaked a Napoleon. The pastry didn't taste as wonderful as she remembered. But things had gone past mere taste. She was trying for one of life's great pleasures: proving her doctor wrong. Half expecting her head to explode, she lingered in the washroom. "You see, nothing happened," she thought as she looked in the mirror. On the way back to join her husband, she had a second pastry.

It wasn't until the chauffeur was driving them home that Mrs. Rinaldi confessed to her husband what she had done.

"We'll have a great New Year's Day!" he said sarcastically.

She told him not to worry. She felt great.

The grandmother and grandaddy of all giant headaches struck Mrs. Rinaldi at five in the morning. As if Mother Nature were trying to impart an unforgettable message, her trouble didn't stop with a headache. Miserably, she alternated between diarrhea and throwing up.

Unable to take medication by mouth, she had to go into the hospital for three days. But she learned her lesson. During the year and a half I kept in touch with Mrs. Rinaldi, she ate no more foods made with wheat, had no headaches—and *she kept her slender figure.*

Another Dawning

A realization about weight reduction struck me one Sunday morning while reading the *New York Times*. The article reviewing books on weight reduction told how each plan was either dangerous or ineffective. Moreover, only one percent of the patients who lost weight kept their weight down.

Without any effort, my weight had fallen to 176 pounds *and stayed there.* Once she got off the food that was incompatible, Mary Lou's weight had normalized. The same had happened to Mrs. Rinaldi.

Most important of all: we had easily maintained our slender figures.

I began watching my other hefty patients more carefully. I soon realized that if they stayed away from the foods that gave them medical problems and ate foods which were compatible with their chemistry, every overweight patient trimmed down.

My patients and I were on our way to an important discovery: certain incompatible carbohydrates (usually grains, nuts, milk products, beans or table sugar) make many people lose control of their eating and cause them to gain weight. Later I learned that environmental chemicals from things like perfume or gas from the kitchen stove can sometimes knock out people's ability to control their eating.

After sorting out my ideas about incompatibilities and overweight, I began visiting medical libraries to learn whether other doctors had observed the connection.

Prominent Physicians Agree

Theron Randolph, M.D., who was once an instructor in medicine at the same medical school where I was on the faculty (Northwestern

University School of Medicine in Chicago), years ago published a scientific paper on the subject.

Dr. Randolph, Dr. Herbert J. Rinkel of the University of Oklahoma Medical School and Dr. Michael Zeller of the University of Illinois School of Medicine, in a disgracefully neglected book, *Food Allergy*, said that certain incompatible foods made people overweight.

The late Dr. Arthur F. Coca, Professor of Clinical Medicine at Columbia University and one of the world's prominent immunologists who wrote many scientific papers as well as a textbook on immunology, maintained that food incompatibilities caused most weight problems.

None of these physicians, however, realized that "new" foods (those foods added to mankind's diet in significant amounts only during the last 5000 to 10,000 years) are the foods that most commonly result in incompatibilities and excess weight. The other doctors did not understand that incompatibilities cause spree eating and they didn't classify overweight patients as *Type-A* or *Type-B*.

3

New Foods Versus Old Foods: Evolution Helps Us Understand Our Weight Problems

Life is a chemical reaction.
—ANTOINE LAVOISIER

Have We Conquered Nature?

We love our technical playthings. We glory in the feeling of power we get from speeding a two-ton, air-conditioned automobile along a superhighway. We delight in jetting across the Atlantic in three hours aboard the Concorde. When we watch an astronaut leap about in the moon dust, we marvel at our cleverness.

We love the products of our technology because they make us feel that we are a part of a wonderful new scientific age. Machines make us believe that we are all-powerful. Our gadgets have contributed to our most cherished delusion, the delusion that says we are above the Laws of Nature.

If you think about it, however, you'll realize that we can put a person on the moon only if we obey every Law of Nature. Break just one law and the spaceship explodes in a fiery disaster and falls into the drink.

For some reason man dislikes seeing himself as a part of the animal kingdom. Man hates to admit that, like all animals, he too is subjected to the laws of evolution and biochemistry. It makes him feel weak, as if he is not in control.

19

To lose weight we must accept our biology. We are biological creatures who must observe the Laws of Nature. Before we can follow the laws, however, we need to understand them. That's what this book's about.

Evolution Helps Us Understand

I have discovered that the "new" foods which have been added to mankind's diet within the last 5,000 to 10,000 years are the foods most likely to cause weight problems and other troubles. These new foods (grains, sugar, milk and milk products) are the foods I find most likely to be incompatible with our biochemistries. Illnesses caused by eating the new foods extend all the way from arthritis, to high blood pressure, to lupus—and far beyond. The same new foods cause both *Type-A* and *Type-B* weight problems.

Why? Because evolution has not yet had enough time to change the chemistry of all of us to efficiently handle the new foods.

We are accustomed to seeing people with short, turned-up noses and people with long, arched noses. Walk down any street and you'll pass some people who are six feet, four inches tall and others only five feet.

Because we cannot see people's biochemistries, however, we forget that each person has a different set of biochemical machinery. Biochemical variation is much greater than physical variation. If we could see people's biochemistry in terms of height, some people would be one inch tall and others 16 feet tall.

Considering the great variations in human chemistry, it's not surprising that some people can handle one food and others need a very different food. Think of the nursery rhyme:

> *Jack Sprat could eat no fat*
> *And his wife could eat no lean.*

Suppose you inherited a race horse that had just won the Kentucky Derby. Furthermore, let's say you happened to have a cattle ranch and therefore had a ready supply of cheap meat. What would happen if you decided to feed your horse beef rather than oats?

Your first problem: The horse would not eat the meat. He has been accustomed to eating oats. He enjoys eating oats.

After thinking over the problem, you decide to grind the meat into oatsize pellets. You then cook up an oat sauce and pour it over the meat pellets and thus actually get your horse to eat meat.

You would find that your horse developed excessive gas, that his eyes had a depressed, hung-over expression, and that he was always tired. In spite of his sad experience, you decide he only needs to go back to the track and get into the spirit and excitement of a race.

Your horse comes in last.

"No wonder he lost," the trainer tells you. "I've been trying to make you understand that your horse doesn't feel good. You're feeding him meat. That's all wrong for him. If he's ever going to win another race, you've got to feed him oats."

"I don't understand why," you say. "I eat meat and I feel great on it."

"Look, meat might be right for you, but everybody knows that horses do well on oats. Horses have been eating oats forever."

You take the trainer's advice, feed your horse oats and he starts to look magnificent. His dull coat and sad eyes turn bright. His step becomes light and energetic. He is again in high spirits. Now he actually enjoys his workouts. You enter him in a race and he wins.

The trainer must have been right: Horses perform better when they eat oats.

Why?

Horses, and the ancestors of the modern horse, are known to have lived on the plains and eaten grasses and seeds for more than 50 million years. The forces of evolution—a process of natural selection that allows the survival of the fittest—designed the horse's biochemical machinery to efficiently handle the foods available to it.

By selective breeding, we might well come up with a strain of horses that could thrive on meat. That task, however, might require a million years to complete. You simply cannot change overnight a biochemistry that has been molded for grain-eating for 50 million years.

Four million years ago mankind's distant ancestors lived in the tropical rain forests and ate fruit as their main source of food. The worldwide drought that occurred during the late Miocene era shrank the rain forests. With the shrinkage of the rain forests, our ancestors' traditional food supply of fruit also shrank. The shortage of food forced our ancestors to leave the forests and begin seeking food on the grass-lands. Grazing animals such as antelopes and buffalo lived on the grass. The grazing animals became our ancestors' new source of food.

A little over two million years ago, meat and animal fat had become our ancestors' most important source of food. Thus for 2.2 million years evolution altered and fine-honed our biochemistry to efficiently use a large amount of meat and animal fat for fuel.

I constantly run into people who have grossly distorted notions about man's early diet. The information in this book about early diets has been reviewed and approved by Edward T. Hall, Ph.D., Professor of Anthropology, Emeritus, Northwestern University. As an anthropolo-gist, he is an authority on early man. His views on mankind's early diet are shared by almost all anthropologists.

The Würm Glaciation

Evolution further molded and specialized our meat and animal fat handling biochemistry during the Würm glaciation when gleaming sheets of ice covered much of northern Europe. The glaciation lasted 65,000 years and ended only about 12,000 years ago. The parts of Europe not covered by glaciers were as cold as a refrigerator. Trees and bushes disappeared. A tough grass was about the only vegetation left. The animals ate the grass, and the people ate the animals. The animals, along with a very few plants, were all our European ancestors had available to eat.

Prior to the Würm glaciation, evolution had altered the chemistry of our ancestors' bodies to best handle a fish-fowl-meat-raw vegetable-raw fruit diet.

During the Würm glaciation, people with biochemistries that could not work well on a fish-fowl-meat diet simply sickened and died. Thus, through the force of evolution, the fish-fowl-meat handling chemical machinery of our ancestors was perfected even more and passed on to us.

Because our European ancestors gradually learned to make better weapons and thus became more efficient hunters, they thrived and reproduced in ever greater numbers. Their efficiency, however, brought about another problem: They began to kill so many of the large animals that meat and fat were no longer available in the amounts needed to feed the expanding population. That happened about 12,000 years ago, a mere half a tick of the clock in terms of evolutionary time.

Fortunately, the shortage of meat occurred at the end of the Würm glaciation, when the ice began receding and Europe once again started enjoying warm sunshine and a milder climate. Our ancestors had to choose between growing food, migrating or starving. Gradually they turned to animal husbandry and agriculture for food.

The new foods—grains, milk, nuts and beans—began to assume an important place in their diet. This change occurred about 10,000 years ago around the Mediterranean. Later, about 5,000 years ago, people in northern Europe began eating the new foods.

One of the newest foods of all, table sugar, appeared in significant amounts only about 150 years ago.

Some people can eat all the wheat and sugar they want and not become ill or overweight. Evolution has adapted their chemistry to handle the new foods. Many of us, however, still have a primitive biochemistry that evolution has not changed enough to deal with the new foods.

We think of evolution as something that happened a long time ago to funny-looking hairy men and women. Not so. Evolution continues altering us. Today evolution operates on Park Avenue just as surely as in the dark rain forests of Africa.

Time and evolution will slowly change mankind's body chemistry so that everyone will live in peace with the new foods. That time, however, is thousands of years in the future. Meanwhile, to stay healthy—and to keep our weight normal—many of us must eat the old foods that better suit the old-fashioned biochemistry we've inherited.

If you are overweight, if you suffer from any illness—from chronic fatigue to depression to gastrointestinal problems—the chances are that the new grain-sugar-milk diet is incompatible with your biochemistry. What your doctor calls illness is usually a sign that evolution is trying to remove your genes from mankind's genetic pool.

If you're overweight, evolution is surely trying to eliminate you. Overweight people are more inclined than slender people to develop many illnesses, all the way from diabetes to high blood pressure and cancer.

And think about this: If you're overweight you'll have more trouble finding a mate, you'll be less fertile and have fewer children, you'll experience more difficulty advancing in your work, you'll find it harder to dodge a speeding car. You'll be the last to escape a burning building. If you require surgery, you have a smaller chance of surviving it. A mugger will see you as easy prey. If he attacks you, you will not be able to escape by running away, and you will be a less likely to fight him off successfully.

Evolution wants to eliminate you and your genes—and me and my genes.

Beat The System

Just as rocket engineers have learned to circumvent the force of gravity, *I've discovered how to outwit the force of evolution. You too will know how it's done when you finish reading this book.*

The human mind made the food-threatening world in which we now live.

Your mind—guided by this book—can show you how to free yourself from the trap that makes you overweight.

Like painting the bedroom or building a patio, losing weight is a project. It takes planning, time and effort.

Losing weight is the most important project you'll ever undertake. Losing weight can save your life. Perhaps even more important, losing weight will surely give you a better life and help you get more of the things you want from life.

4

The Appestat Explains *Type-A* Weight Problems: The Spree Eater

The laws of Nature are so simple, we have to rise above the complexity of scientific thought to see them.

—RICHARD FEYNMAN

RUTH ANDERSON

A beautiful woman with a centerfold figure, a stage and screen star had been the toast of the country until she lost control of her eating and packed on 42 extra pounds. We'll call her Ruth Anderson. Because of her excess weight, she lost starring roles. Directors would only use her for character parts. Her income plunged and with it went her feeling of self-worth.

Ruth was hungry all the time. Somehow she would force herself to stay on a tight, calorie-counted diet day after day and, worse, night after night. Now and then, however, she would turn uncontrollably hungry. She would rage inside until she feared something would snap and she would do something bizarre like tearing off her clothes and running nude through the streets of New York.

"I hate myself!" she said on her first visit to my office. She actually struck herself on the hips. "Look at me. I'm a pig!"

Weeping, she took a frayed-about-the-edges photograph from her purse and handed it to me.

"That's how I looked only two-and-a-half years ago."

25

The photograph showed a sylph-slender, laughing beach beauty in a bikini tossing a Frisbee.

"It will shock you when I tell you about my eating sprees," she said.

"I don't shock easily."

This confession was difficult for her. She breathed in and out several times.

In addition to scuba-diving equipment, she had decided to give her nephew something personal for his birthday. She would bake him an apple pie. The pie had not finished baking before she realized she had made a poor choice. The delicious odor of the hot pie made her hungry.

She began pacing the floor and drinking a diet soda. To distract herself, she switched on the TV. She sipped black coffee that was hot enough—she hoped—to burn away her hunger.

When the pie finished cooking, she leaned down to inhale its wonderful aroma. One of the strips of pastry hung over the edge, spoiling the perfection of her culinary creation. She broke off the end of the strip. Before she realized what she was doing, she put the crust in her mouth and ate it.

Within three minutes her hunger increased so sharply that she began to feel wild and disorganized. Her insides churned. She was ready to kill for something to eat—specifically, for anything made of wheat and sugar. She pulled her coat from the closet and rushed out the front door. At the corner deli her hands shook as she paid for a small bag of cookies. She tore open the bag and shoved one into her mouth as she began hurrying down a side street. She prayed no one would recognize her. She dug dark glasses from her coat pocket.

She finished the cookies and stopped at an ice cream shop. Only one pint. One pint of tutti-frutti and then absolutely no more. She promised herself that she would make three extra trips to her exercise class this week to work off the extra calories. Two more bags of cookies and three quarts of ice cream later, Ruth returned to her apartment.

She looked at her face in the mirror and screamed, "You pig, I hate you!" And then she ate the birthday pie! In tears she threw herself down on the bed and buried her face in her pillow.

After she finished telling me her story she asked, "Can you help somebody like me?"

"I can help you if you'll cooperate."

"Just tell me what to do."

"First, under controlled conditions you must eat certain foods, leave them off and eat them again so we can learn about your particular biochemistry. We need to learn which foods are compatible and which are incompatible with your biochemistry. You might need to make some adjustments in your environment."

"Do I have to cook the food?"

"Testing is simpler if you do the cooking."

"But I don't know how to cook."

"Cooking's very simple. I'll tell you how."

"But I can't do it this month. Edgar, one of my boyfriends from the coast, is coming to New York and Edgar likes to eat at all the best restaurants."

"It's entirely up to you."

My answer turned her off. She wanted me to beg.

Ruth returned a month later—after having gained seven pounds. I don't know why she came back. This time she had to put off losing weight because she was jetting to France to appear in a movie. She would be back in six weeks. On and on it went, excuse after excuse.

"Why waste your money and my time?" I finally asked her.

"Oh, but I do want to lose weight. I'm deadly serious about it."

"Then become involved. Show up here every week and get on the scales."

"I will, just as soon as I finish a commercial in Florida. I absolutely promise."

"It's your life and your career. I'm here to help you, but I can't do it for you."

She returned once again. Overflowing with tears, she told me how Edgar had called her a fat slob and dropped her. Her agent threatened to release her if she didn't lose 40 pounds.

Ruth never got started on my program. I see her on a talk show now and then or in minor movie rolls. She's fatter than ever. One of her friends tells me she's always either high on drugs or so depressed she can talk about nothing except killing herself.

Your eating sprees—your *Type-A* problem—might not be as dramatic as Ruth's, but you get the idea.

Warning!

The apple tart that the actress *only smelled and tasted* set off a reaction that sent her on an eating spree. I've had patients simply walk past a bakery, *smell the wheat,* and go on an eating spree.

Remember, you can detect an odor only if particles of the substance are in the air. When you smell something, particles have entered your body. They quickly enter your body chemistry by penetrating the mucous membranes of your nose and lungs.

Spree Drinkers, Spree Eaters

Alcoholics (spree drinkers) have one drink and then another and another until they reach the end of their drinking spree. Alcoholism is actually one form of food incompatibility.

The spree eater also loses control, but instead of drinking, he or she eats.

The Appetite-Control Center

Are you tired of staying indoors? Would you like to laugh through the latest Eddie Murphy movie playing at a theater at Third Avenue and 59th Street? Your brain will tell you whether you have the time and money. If the answer is "yes," your brain will remind you that it's cold outside. Then your brain will take over and direct your muscles so you can put on your coat, and go through all the steps needed for you to walk to the corner. Your brain will then help you decide whether to shoot a hand up and hail a taxi, or do your body a favor and walk.

In short, our *brains* help us take charge of our bodies and control our interactions with other people and with the world around us.

Do you work too hard? Suppose you were a buyer for Bloomingdale's and had 15 minutes to select a hundred watches to add to the stock, then decide on 200 earrings and 300 bracelets.

What if at the same time you were buying the things for the store you also had to remember to breathe 16 times a minute, to make your heart beat 74 times a minute, to perspire if your body temperature started climbing, and to stop perspiring when your body temperature began falling?

Too many tasks at one time would make you frustrated and careless. You would pick the wrong watches, forget to breathe, or allow yourself to be distracted from the boring task of regulating your body temperature.

Automatic control centers in our brains handle most of our routine physical functions. Automatic control centers take care of tasks like the regulation of body temperature and breathing. In the primitive part of the brain known as the hypothalamus we find the automatic appetite control center known as the *appestat.*

Appestat is not a catchy Madison-Avenue word that I've dreamed up. If you will stop by the library and read page 839 in the latest (11th) edition of the textbook on physiology most commonly used in medical schools, *Best and Taylor's Physiological Basis of Medical Practice,* you can read for yourself many of the known facts about the appestat.

Why isn't the appestat mentioned more often? Practicing physicians ignore many facts in textbooks. No one teaches them how to properly apply nutritional information to help them care for their patients.

Knowledge about your appestat, however, can change your life. First, you need to know that two types of cells make up the appestat: the *turn-on* cells, and the *turn-off* cells.

The Turn-On *Cells*

One group of cells (nuclei) makes us hungry. They initiate our desire to eat. For that reason I call them the *turn-on* cells.

"Eat! Eat! Eat!" they urge us all during our waking hours. "Keep on eating more, more, more!" The full-time job of these *turn-on* cells is to make us hungry.

Researchers have deliberately damaged the *turn-on* cells in experimental animals. After damaging the *turn-on* cells, nothing tells the animal to eat. Unless force-fed, the animal will starve.

If our *turn-on* cells are healthy and constantly urge us to eat, why don't we eat all the time?

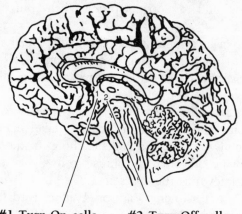

#1 Turn-On cells.   #2 Turn-Off cells.

The Turn-Off Cells

We have a second group of cells in our appetite-control center. I call them the *turn-off* cells.

The *turn-off* cells hold the *turn-on* cells in check. If something damages our *turn-off* cells, nothing tells us to stop eating. We continue eating like a machine that's lost its governor. We become overweight.

Here's a cutaway illustration of the human brain showing the location of the *turn-on* and *turn-off* cells in the appestat center.

Appestat Control Center in the Brain

Scientists at Johns Hopkins and other medical centers have used instruments to damage the *turn-off* cells. They did experiments on mice, rats, cats, dogs and monkeys. When they damaged the *turn-off* cells, nothing told the animals that they had eaten enough. They ate extra food and grew fat.

Chemical Damage

Researchers at Harvard injected the chemical phlorhizin into the brains of experimental animals near the *turn-off* cells. These injections *temporarily* damaged the *turn-off* cells and *temporarily* increased hunger.

Scientists at the National Institutes of Health and in the U.S. Army Medical Department injected a chemical called goldthioglucose. That chemical also *temporarily* damaged the appestat's *turn-off* cells.

After repeated temporary damage to the *turn-off* cells and the resulting periods of overeating, the animals became fat.

The medical profession agrees that certain medications, such as tranquilizers, damage the *turn-off* cells. This damage causes patients to eat too much and gain weight.

Brain damage, whether from viral infections or injuries, can harm the *turn-off* cells and make people overweight. (The condition, however, is *extremely* rare. Don't try to get off the hook by blaming your overeating on brain damage.)

The late Dr. Roger Williams at the University of Texas collected evidence that vitamin deficiencies can damage the appestat cells as well.

A team of doctors working at Columbia University showed that lack of enough protein in the mother's diet during pregnancy can harm a child's appestat. The result is an overweight child.

If you are overweight and want to become slim again, the news that vitamin and mineral deficiencies, deficiencies in protein, and that certain chemicals can damage turn-off cells should excite you. Especially if you're a spree eater and suffer from Type-A weight problems.

Because only certain chemicals can damage the *turn-off* cells in the brain, this means that *turn-off* cells are different from all other cells in the body. Chemicals like goldthioglucose do not damage the cells in the big toe or the cells in the tongue or the cells in the brain that control breathing.

Research showing that chemicals can selectively damage the turn-off cells in the appestat helps explain how you can lose control of your hunger and become overweight.

My Theory

If we suffer from *Type-A* weight problems (spree eating), it means that we have trouble with our *turn-off* cells. Our *turn-off* cells don't tell us to stop eating. They fail to shout, "Stop! You've had enough!"

Ice cream makes many people want to go on an eating spree. From my patients I've learned that different foods make different people uncontrollably hungry. *Always, however, it's one of the new foods that blasts people into the eating-spree orbit.*

When we eat, particles of food escape digestion and enter our bloodstreams directly. These small bits of food temporarily are toxic to the *turn-off* cells and damage them. Once the *turn-off* cells are damaged and cannot function properly, nothing tells people to stop eating. They go on wild eating sprees. The foods are incompatible with their chemistry.

I've concluded that *spree eaters have their turn-off cells temporarily damaged by one or more of the "new" foods. When damaged, turn-off cells are unable to function. They don't tell people when to stop eating. The damage is temporary. It's the same type of damage caused by goldthioglucose and phlorhizin in laboratory animals.*

Later I'll tell you how environmental substances (like formaldehyde from new carpeting, or cat dander) can also knock out the appestat cells and cause Type-A obesity.

People who have their *turn-off* cells knocked out don't die from the condition, so I have no autopsy material to back up my theory. If, however, someone did die in the middle of an eating spree, I suspect a microscopic examination of the *turn-off* cells in their appestat center would show cells that were badly swollen. Those swollen cells would not be able to work properly. The appestat center wouldn't be able to shout, "Stop!" when they had enough to eat.

Evidence

1. By exposing patients to suspected foods, I can bring on hunger in those who suffer from *Type-A* weight problems.
2. I have taken careful clinical histories on *Type-A* patients. They feel desperately hungry after eating certain foods, almost always one of the foods that's new to the human diet.

Questionnaire To Help Identify a *Type-A* Weight Problem

1. Do you continue eating after your hunger should be satisfied?
2. Do you enjoy eating until you feel a loaded, stretched, heavy sensation in your stomach?
3. Do you sneak food after eating a regular meal with other people?
4. Do you lose control so you are unable to stop eating?
5. Do you feel more hungry after eating?
6. Would you be ashamed to tell other people how much you eat?
7. Do you eat rapidly even when you're not in a hurry?
8. Would you sometimes be willing to spend almost any amount of money for food?

If you're overweight and your answer is yes to any of the above questions, then you have a *Type-A* weight problem.

Earlier in the book we spoke briefly about addictive eaters. In the next chapter we'll explore in more depth the world of the addictive eater. Remember, the addictive eater is the person who feels compelled to eat a *certain* food. They suffer from *Type-B* weight problems.

5

Chocoholics, Cookie Munchers, and Other *Type-B* Addictive Eaters

Discovery consists in seeing what everybody else has seen and thinking what nobody has thought.
—ALBERT SZENT-GYÖRGYI

"**C**hocolate! I'm afraid I'm addicted to chocolate."

"I don't feel right unless I have a dessert after dinner."

"I can't get started in the morning without my sweet roll and coffee."

People who make such statements are addicted. If overweight, they're suffering from a *Type-B* weight problem, addictive eating. They need to repeatedly eat a certain food to protect themselves from unpleasant withdrawal symptoms.

JACK JOHNSON

Jack Johnson had to eat something sweet after every meal; otherwise, he would develop a headache, irritability and depression. One night Jack had dinner on a flight from Seattle to Chicago. The airline ran out of desserts. He missed his sugar fix.

Jack arrived at the airport in the middle of withdrawal from sugar: he felt irritable, depressed, and had a "tension" headache. Jack exploded and nearly started a fight when a man accidentally jostled him. He knew

34

something was wrong. He didn't realize just what was bothering him until he passed a snack bar and saw a family eating chocolate sundaes.

I didn't have my dessert! he suddenly remembered.

He went inside and ordered pecan pie à la mode. Three minutes after he finished the pie he began to relax. His headache vanished and again he felt at peace with the world.

Eating sugar masked Jack's sugar withdrawal symptoms. (Let's be thankful that Jack wasn't piloting the plane. In the midst of a sugar withdrawal reaction he might have forgotten to check the fuel gauge— and wham! evolution would eliminate him and his genes!)

Reinforced Behavior

Because Jack felt better after eating a sweet, the experience reinforced his sugar-eating behavior. Eating sugar rewarded him. He lost his unpleasant withdrawal symptoms.

Gradually, Jack became conditioned—like one of Pavlov's dogs— by a pain-pleasure response.

Addictions usually grow worse. When Jack suffered from withdrawal symptoms, he got his reward each time he ate sugar. Thus he continued his sugar eating at shorter and shorter intervals. He upped his caloric intake and added unwanted pounds. Jack was a typical addictive eater and suffered from a *Type-B* weight problem.

Motivated and bright, right away Jack caught on to the logic of my system. When he traveled, he began taking his secretary to cook for him so he could properly test his foods.

He lost his bulging-fat stomach. His secretary went on the same diet and watched her cellulite disappear. The last I heard from Jack, he sent me a wedding announcement and enclosed a note. He was marrying his secretary. They had moved to L.A.

Addictions Control Many Lives

Addictions are among the strongest forces motivating mankind. The drive for the addictive substance (whether for bread, candy bars, cheesecake, cigarettes, alcohol or heroin) is stronger than the drive for fame and money, stronger even than the drive for sex, and often stronger than the drive for life itself. Many addicted people do not hesitate to risk their lives for a fix. An overweight man with high blood pressure keeps eating sweets. A three-pack-a-day cigarette smoker continues courting lung cancer. A heroin addict risks his life in a holdup to get the money for just one more fix.

My Addictions

During my fat years I was addicted to ice cream. It sounds very American, doesn't it? That's because America is a country of overweight people. If we're addicted to a "food" that contains granular sugar (like candy) or a grain (like cake, corn muffins or sweet rolls), the chances are that we'll be overweight.

I'm still addicted. Almost everyone in the modern world is addicted. It happens, however, that *I've changed my addictions to a non-fattening food*. Nowadays I'm addicted to coffee, which leaves no calories in its wake. I keep telling myself that I'm going to stop coffee just as soon as I finish writing the book I'm working on. Maybe I will. Maybe I won't. I told myself the same thing while writing my last book. Maybe I always start a new book on the day I finish my old one so I'll always have an excuse to postpone dropping my last addiction. Like you, I'm very fond of the thing to which I'm addicted.

♦ *coffee drinkers beware: Coffee may knock out your appestat and make you hungry, thus coffee may indirectly make you add weight.*
♦ Never drink low-calorie diet sodas. They are disasters. Tests have proven that people who drink diet sodas gain weight. I find diet drinks quite toxic for my patients. Often the drinks knock out their appestats and make them hungry.
♦ Juices are also disasters for those who want to lose weight.
♦ As I will detail later, people who want to lose weight will fail if they drink alcoholic beverages.

Fate has cast me in the role of a "puller." I spend much of my time trying to pull people off of their addictive foods like bread and cake and bialys and ice cream. Need I tell you that mine is a difficult life?

When I'm reincarnated, I hope I come back as a pusher rather than a puller. It's much easier to earn a living pushing cigarettes, or ice cream, or chocolate bars than trying to pull people away from such addictions.

Many common foods ("new" foods) are just as addictive as heroin. Some of them are as dangerous—possibly more so. If you are addicted to a carbohydrate (wheat and sugar are the two biggest ones), the chances are you're overweight and that your addiction will shorten your life.

The chances are also very good that the food to which you're addicted is incompatible with your biochemistry and that it gives you problems other than obesity.

A housewife from Saddle River, New Jersey consulted me because of a high blood pressure problem. By manipulating her diet, I discovered that a wheat incompatibility triggered her high blood pressure.

"Can I have just one piece of toast every morning?" she asked.

"I don't know, but I know how to find out."

She ate one piece of toast every morning for a week and returned for a blood pressure check. It had shot up again. She had her answer.

Don't forget: It's the food you like best (and the person you like best) that gives you the most trouble.

Because a food to which you are addicted often harms you in some way, your addiction may prevent you from realizing your full potential as a human being. For example, if I eat wheat at night and start to write the next morning, I'll have trouble gathering my ideas and combining them properly on paper. That's because wheat is incompatible with my brain chemistry. Wheat interferes with the metabolism of my brain cells and makes them work less efficiently. If I ate wheat regularly, I'm certain my I.Q. would drop 20 points. I don't know about you, but I haven't got 20 points to throw away.

I often wonder what percentage of school dropouts would finish school if they ate no grains, table sugar or milk or milk products. I would guess that the dropout rate would fall by at least 50 percent.

Here's how the World Health Organization characterizes drug addicts:

1. Addicts have an overpowering desire to take a drug.
2. They will get the drug any way possible.
3. They usually increase their intake of the drug.
4. They develop a psychological and a physical dependency on the drug.

Substitute the word "food" for "drug" in the above definition and you'll understand food addictions.

I would like to remind you that the narcotic addict must have his narcotic (his "fix") at regular intervals if he is to avoid withdrawal symptoms. So it is with the food addict.

Like the heroin addict, the person with a *Type-B* weight problem must eat his addictive food to avoid withdrawal symptoms.

Understanding Food Addiction

At the University of Kyoto in Japan, several scientists grew chicken embryo tissue in a nutrient "soup" that contained morphine.

As a second step in the experiment, they transferred the cells to a soup free of morphine. The cells grown in the solution containing the morphine had become accustomed to the morphine, had incorporated the morphine as a part of their cellular chemistry. The cells had become addicted.

When the researchers removed the cells from the soup containing the morphine, the cells had withdrawal symptoms. The cells became ill. The longer the cells lived with the morphine, the more striking was their withdrawal damage.

How did the scientists discover the cell damage?

For one thing, the cells stopped reproducing. Also, when they examined the cells under a microscope, they found the cells twisted and drawn. The cells showed other marked signs of physical degeneration. Had these cells belonged to a living animal, they could not have carried out their normal functions.

When the scientists gave the withdrawal-sick cells morphine, the cells regained their normal rate of growth and took on their usual healthy appearance.

Please don't quote me as saying that morphine improves your health. I simply want to point out that when the scientists suddenly withdrew morphine from morphine-addicted cells, the cells became ill. They "cured" (masked) the withdrawal illness by giving them morphine once more.

Conclusion: Living cells exposed to morphine incorporate morphine into their chemistry. Morphine becomes essential to their chemistry. Thus the cells need morphine—as they also need food and water—for good health.

Withdraw the morphine and you take away a chemical essential to the cells' chemistry. The cells get sick. Add the morphine once more, and the cells recover from the withdrawal illness.

The morphine masked the symptoms brought on by withdrawal.

If morphine is permantely withdrawn, after four days the cellular chemistry readjusts on a new level and begins functioning normally again in spite of the absence of morphine.

So it appears to be with foods. Certain new foods may become a part of the body chemistry. If the addictive food is eliminated, patients suffer withdrawal symptoms for about four days. Then their biochemistry settles down and returns to normal.

The reason most Type-B overweight patients fail to lose weight *is that they are not willing to suffer through the withdrawal phase of weight loss.*

The reason most Type-B overweight patients regain *their lost weight is that they become readdicted.* As with heroin, morphine and other narcotics, it is very easy to become readdicted to certain foods.

People with food addictions have a food (or a breakdown product of a food) become a part of their cellular chemistry. When they remove the food, their chemistry is *temporarily* disrupted.

After removing the addictive food, people with food addictions are ill (some more, some less) for three or four days.

If people eat the addictive food during the withdrawal period, the withdrawal symptoms disappear. Eating the addictive food "masks" the symptoms.

New Foods vs. Old Foods

I see exceptions, but *generally* the old foods—foods such as *fresh* fish-fowl-meat-*fresh raw* low-carbohydrate vegetables-*fresh raw* low carbohydrate fruits—that our ancestors have been eating for more than two million years are not addictive for the patients who consult me. (Often carrots and fruits—especially sweet fruits—are an exception. To increase sales, I suspect that agriculturists have developed them so they contain more sugar than they did in the original wild state.)

Generally, it's the new foods which not only make us overweight but cause a great many of mankind's illness such as headaches, ulcers, backaches, lupus, adult-onset diabetes, arthritis, asthma and a host of other diseases.

Combined Type-A and Type-B

Many people are not pure *Type-A* or *Type-B*. Often they are a combination of the two. Sometimes people are a *Type-A* for a few months and later become a *Type-B*, or the other way around.

BILL WATSON

Bill Watson visited my office the other day. His chief complaint was a history of obesity dating back to childhood. Now at age 42, his family doctor told him he had high blood pressure and needed to lose 80 pounds. When Bill visited me he put his problem bluntly:

"I'm convinced that if I don't lose weight I'm going to die while I'm still middle-aged."

Bill suffered from both *Type-A* and *Type-B* obesity. He liked to go on eating sprees. Ice cream was his passion. One day he ate 26 different flavors of ice cream. Still not satisfied, he got in his car and headed for more ice cream stores. He found them closed. That didn't stop him. He sped through the Lincoln Tunnel onto the Jersey Turnpike and cruised around half the night stopping at turnpike food shops for more ice cream.

He was a spree eater. He suffered from a *Type-A* weight problem. A night of spree eating, however, didn't keep him away from his regular addiction the next day. Bill was addicted to a sugary cola drink. As a commercial artist, he sat all day at a drawing board with a large bottle of his sugar-charged cola drink resting in a wire basket hanging nearby. On an average day he would empty three giant-size bottles of soda.

"My hands shake and my mind won't work right if I don't have my cola," he told me.

Decidedly, Bill suffered from both a *Type-A* and *Type-B* weight problem.

The going was rough. For months Bill would start and stop his diet. *Persistence is the horse that wins.* Finally, he discovered leaving off the foods—and drinks!—that made him overweight left him with an entirely different personality. The foods that were incompatible with his chemistry had been having a sedative (toxic) effect on him. Without his sugary drink he simply could not sit at a drawing board all day. He got a position as art director for an ad agency. The job allowed him much more freedom to move around. He learned to burn up his drive rather than sedate it with foods that made him toxic. Incidentally, by "burning" his energy instead of sedating it with toxic foods, he increased his income.

"My God!" he said one day. "Who would believe that Bill Watson would ever join a gym?"

After losing weight, he began dating. Much to his surprise, women were interested in him. He discovered he had a natural sense of rhythm that made him a good dancer.

Questionnaire to Help Identify *Type-B* Weight Problems

1. Do you often yearn for a particular food?
2. Do you feel dissatisfied unless you eat a certain food?
3. Do you suffer any of these symptoms before eating: weakness, tiredness, headache, restlessness, depression, irritability?
4. Do the above symptoms disappear after you eat?
5. Will you go out of your way to locate a certain food that you crave?
6. Do you daydream about eating a particular food?
7. Do you stock up on one or two particular foods to make certain you always have a good supply?
8. Do you buy books on how to cook a certain food—bread, for example?
9. Are you dissatisfied unless you finish a meal with something sweet?
10. Are you well-known among your friends for a certain type of recipe?

If you are overweight and your answer to any of the above questions is yes, you are suffering from a *Type-B* weight problem.

As mentioned, many people have mied *Type-A* and *Type-B* weight problems. They suffer from both spree eating and addictive eating. In a pure *Type-B*, we find no spree eating.

6

Vitamins and Other Supplements You Need for Weight Loss

Vitamins, if properly understood and applied, will help us to reduce human suffering to an extent which the most fantastic mind would fail to imagine.

—ALBERT SZENT-GYÖRGYI

Sunshine and desert warmth greeted me in Palm Springs, California when I arrived to speak at a meeting called to celebrate the 50th anniversary of Albert Szent-Györgyi's discovery of chemically pure crystalline vitamin C. Age 85, eyes twinkling, still full of humor, Szent-Györgyi could have stopped by Universal Studios on his way to Palm Springs to be made-up and costumed to play the part of the grand old man of science, a Nobel Laureate. He had shaggy hair, a furrowed face and mismatched baggy jacket and trousers. Even if the president of the United States had been attending the meeting, however, Szent-Györgyi would have dominated the room.

"Now that all of you know I'm civilized enough to own a tie and jacket, I'm going to take them off," he said before beginning his speech.

Strange twists and quirks of chance litter the field of every scientific discovery, especially so in the case of Szent-Györgyi's discovery of ascorbic acid, which, while working on it, he called "Godnose."

A struggling, church-mouse poor student in Wisconsin probably discovered vitamin C in the early 1920s. His tight-fisted dean refused to give him a grant of a few hundred dollars to scientifically prove what he had found.

In 1925, two U.S. Army scientists isolated vitamin C, but just before they came up with scientific proof, red tape entangled them and transferred them to a different duty. They never completed their work.

A Russian scientist in France probably also isolated the precious crystals in 1925. For some reason he dropped his research before completion. (Who knows why? Maybe he fell in love.)

In 1928, Albert Szent-Györgyi, a Hungarian working at Cambridge on an entirely different project, isolated what he thought was vitamin C. But he had to return to his native country before he could complete the proof. In 1931, Szent-Györgyi picked up the work again and proved his great discovery.

As if throwing dice, immortality chose Szent-Györgyi. The other researchers have long been forgottern.

At the meeting in Palm Springs, Szent-Györgyi bemoaned the trouble he had getting the medical profession to understand vitamin C. After making his discovery, repeatedly doctors asked him, "We already knew how to prevent scurvy. Now that you've discovered pure crystalline vitamin C, what's it good for—other than preventing scurvy?"

Vitamin research fell out of fashion during the 1940s. Not only did Szent-Györgyi fail to get the medical profession to fully understand vitamin C, but even he had difficulty raising money to further his research. The medical profession distressed him. He thought only a small percentage of physicians would ever learn even the bare basics of nutrition.

Good Clinical Advice Is Rare

Sadly, the public still has difficulty getting useful information about vitamins and other nutritional supplements. In the U.S., professors who should understand vitamins often know least of all. They spend their lives working with laboratory animals and usually have little clinical experience treating humans.

As the U.S. *Congressional Record* shows, manufacturers of grain, sugar, and milk products give many professors money for their research, pay their expenses to "scientific" meetings in charming faraway places, and often put them on salary as members of the boards of directors to legally "buy them off" year after year. That is, for as long as the professors are willing to see no evil, hear no evil, speak no evil about the three horsemen of the apoocalypse: grains, sugar and milk.

When senators—or writers, or TV producers—want information about vitamins, they ask the professors, who profess to know, but in reality have little practical knowledge about the very practical subject of nutrition. What information the professors do give out is often colored green—the color of food processors' money.

Do You Need "Extra" Vitamins?

"You get all the vitamins you need from the average American diet."

People who make mail-order statements like that are trying to hide their lack of information.

"If you take extra vitamins, you only lose them in your urine."

True, but until the vitamins are excreted, the body can use them. If we drink extra amounts of water, we only lose it in our urine, yet few people advocate that they drink less water.

For many reasons, each of us should take extra vitamins and other supplements. Losing weight is a stress to the body chemistry. Under stress, the body has higher needs for nutritional supplements.

It's difficult enough to identify and remove the foods from our diet which are incompatible with our individual chemistries. We should not be forced to worry whether we're getting enough vitamins, minerals and unsaturated fats from foods. When we take vitamins and other supplements in adequate amounts, we have one less concern.

We are attacked by food colorings, herbicides, plant-growth regulators, and other antagonists and antimetabolites that enter our food chain. These chemicals constantly bombard our bodies and destroy our enzyme systems. At least dozens—and probably thousands—attack us. Often they attack us by destroying the vitamins in our bodies.

Farmers, for example, commonly use a chemical called maleic hydrazide as a sprout inhibitor for tobacco plants. Traces of the chemical get into tobacco. They enter the body either through smoking or from breathing the air where other people are smoking. Hydrazides are strong vitamin B6 destroyers.

Female sex hormones, birth control pills, some antibiotics, medications for high blood pressure and antidepressants also incapacitate vitamin B6.

Frying and overheating oxidizes fats and oils. Oxidized fats form toxic chemicals that zap vitamin B6. Some people need 200 or more times the official vitamin B6 level, as Leon Rosenberg at Yale has pointed out.

Although I've given a few details about vitamin B6 in particular to illustrate my point, the same principles apply to all vitamins and other supplements.

Another problem is that we can no longer depend upon foods to give us nutrients.

Farmers mass-produce their fruits and vegetables in artificially fertilized, mineral-poor soils. They harvest fruits and vegetables before they ripen. They dip their produce in chemicals and ship it to distant markets. Chicken "manufacturers" turn out chickens whose feet have never touched the ground.

We lose 50 percent of the vitamin B6 when we refine sugar and grains. Canning vegetables and overheating meats also destroy this vitamin.

The simple truth is that we have too many people to feed. The world is badly overpopulated. We are already starving—not for calories, but for food with proper nutrients. I don't know about you, but I haven't eaten a tomato that tasted like a tomato for 20 years.

Individuality

Roger Williams of the University of Texas, Austin, started stressing the chemical individuality of people in the early 1950s.

Since 1968, Nobel Prize-winner Linus Pauling has repeatedly talked and written that vitamin requirements differ from person to person, depending, in part, upon the person's inherited chemical make-up.

When we discover more about individual needs, we'll probably find that each person's ideal vitamin level falls on a bell-shaped curve. Many people who fail to thrive in our society probably fall at the neglected far end of the bell curve.

A vitamin dependency disorder is a chemical defect. Because of the defect, the person suffering from it needs more than the usual amounts of one or more vitamins.

Popular medical textbooks neglect the subject. However, *The Heinz Handbook of Nutrition,* not widely read by physicians, but with a distinguished editorial board, states:

> "The typical individual is more likely to be one who has average needs with respect to many essential nutrients but who also exhibits some nutritional requirements for a few essential nutrients which are far from average."

While waiting for the light to change, people sometimes roll down their car windows and call out questions to me. "What vitamin should I take for my sore shoulder?" or "Will I sleep better if I take calcium?"

Such attitudes irk me. Instead of giving a speech, I wave, smile and continue my walk. Most people do not realize that every cell in the body needs every nutrient. Asking me which vitamin to take for a sore shoulder is like asking the late Leonard Bernstein, "Which note is the most important in Beethoven's Fifth?"

True, you may catch a cold if you lack vitamin C. You may, however, pick up an infection if you have too little vitamin A. We could say the same thing about B complex, zinc, unsaturated fatty acids and others.

Like a symphony, the human body requires every nutrient if it is to work properly.

Will Vitamins Make Me Hungry?

Vitamins will increase your hunger only if:

1. You have a vitamin deficiency that has made you ill, or if
2. You have an incompatibility between your body chemistry and the form of one or more vitamins you take.

Usually, hunger is reduced by taking vitamins and other supplements. The cells of the appestat, like all other cells in the body, cannot work properly unless they are well nourished. The *turn-on* and the *turn-off* cells in the appestat are no exceptions. Unless they are functioning normally, we cannot expect the cells to tell us when to eat and when not to eat. They do their work properly only if we give them vitamins and other nutrients in ideal amounts.

How Much Do We Need?

The naked truth is that no one knows the vitamin and mineral amounts we need. We know, for example, how many milligrams of vitamin C will keep us from dying of scurvy. The problem is, we don't know how much we need to function at our best.

For years the U.S. Government has been telling its citizens that they need 65 mg a day of vitamin C. A scientist working for the government admitted in an article in the *New England Journal of Medicine* ("New Concepts in the Biology of Biochemistry of Ascorbic Acid," 1986) that no one knows the optimum level of vitamin C—or any other vitamin.

I strongly advise you to take added vitamins, minerals and polyunsaturated fats.

I must admit, however, that if you follow a fish-fowl-meat-limited vegetable-limited fruit diet, if you cook the beef rare, if you include beef liver once a week, and if you spend a modest amount of time in the sunlight, you will have a better diet and supply of nutrients than 99 percent of people in the world. The only really disturbing defect in such a diet is an inadequate supply of calcium and magnesium. Those two important minerals are covered later in this chapter.

My strong advice is to take more vitamins and minerals than the body needs. The body discards the excess. Within reason, this works well, though certain limitations must be put on vitamins A, D, E and B6.

"Fast" foods that are short on nutrients make up a large part of the diet of most people with weight problems. Overweight people are more likely than others to have low levels of vitamins, minerals, and unsaturated fats. To attempt weight loss without taking proper supplements is courting trouble and failure.

If you want a terrible program, take one vitamin-mineral tablet a day that "has everything in it." Such tablets will probably keep you from dying from pellagra, but there should be more to life than not dying of pellagra. Believe me, such tablets are the wrong way to go.

Incompatibilities

It's not fair, but it's always possible that any vitamin or other nutritional supplement will disagree with you. Symptoms can vary all the way from headaches to skin rashes, from ordinary gas to stomach cramps and diarrhea. If a vitamin disagrees with you, leave it out for a few days, then try it again. Sometimes it's best to stop all supplements for three or four days, then start them again one at a time.

Often an incompatibility will not show up until you've been taking the vitamin for three or four days. Test the suspected vitamin for three or four days running before deciding whether you're reacting to it.

Once you identify the culprit, try taking a different brand or a different form of the vitamin.

Most people find they tolerate vitamins and other nutritional supplements best if they take them after eating. Remember that your physician should approve of any nutritional supplements you take.

Recommended Supplements

Vitamin A is a fat-soluble vitamin that you must not use in excessive amounts. *Best source*: cod liver oil, one teaspoon daily. (This also contains vitamin D.) As an alternative—but not nearly as health-giving—you can take a natural vitamin A capsule of 10,000 units daily.

Beta-carotene is another form of vitamin A, a pro-vitamin A that the body can turn into vitamin A. You should take beta-carotene along with the vitamin A mentioned above. *Best source*: beta-carotene capsules, 15 mg (25,000 I.U.). One capsule every third day. (NOTE: People trying to lose weight should not eat carrots for carotene. Carrots may either send you on an eating spree or trap you in an addiction.)

Vitamin D is essential for calcium absorption; therefore, it has widespread effects throughout every cell in the body. Vitamin D is another fat-soluble vitamin that can give you trouble if taken in excessive amounts. Best source: cod liver oil, one teaspoon daily (the same cod liver oil suggested above as a source of vitamin A). An alternative is to take a natural vitamin D capsule of 400 units daily.

B Vitamins are a must. The best form is a vitamin B-complex capsule (or tablet) with 50 mg of the major vitamins. Take one after breakfast. Some people feel better if they have a second capsule after lunch. If you take it at night, it might keep you awake.

Here's the composition of the B-complex capsule I often recommend:

Thiamine Mononitrate	50 mg
Riboflavin	50 mg
Pyridoxine HC1	50 mg
Vitamin B12 (cobalamine concentrate)	50 mcg
Niacinamide	50 mg
Pantothenic Acid (calcium pantothenate)	50 mg
Folic Acid	100 mcg
d-Biotin	50 mcg
Inositol	50 mg
Choline Bitartrate	50 mg
Para-aminobenzoic Acid	30 mg

This B-complex capsule has no alfalfa, yeast, etc., as found in many B-complex formulas. Often people are alleregic to alfalfa, yeast, etc.

Even though the B-complex which I recommend is free of most allergenic things, still some people find it troublesome. It's best to start by taking only one-quarter of the capsule daily for four or five days. If all goes well, gradually increase the amount until you take the whole capsule.

How do you take a portion of a capsule? Pull the capsule apart and shake out three-quarters of the powder. Then push the capsule back together again, wipe it off, and swallow it.

Vitamin B6 (pyridoxine) is especially important for the metabolism of proteins. People on a high fish-fowl-meat-vegetable-fruit diet often feel better with extra amounts. *Best source*: Pyridoxine (vitamin B6) capsules 200 mg, one capsule daily. *If you take more than 50 mg a day, remember to stay under the care of a nutritionally knowledgeable physician.*

Vitamin B12, like B6, is needed in extra amounts by many people. Certainly vitamin B12 is especially important for protein metabolism. I have the clinical impression that people taking vitamin B12 find it easier to lose weight. I strongly recommend the *hydroxo*cobalamin (B12b) form of the vitamin rather than the *cyano*cobalamin (B12) form of vitamin B12. The *cyano* form of B12 contains cyanide, a toxic chemical.

Most people do best on B12b injections. Your doctor can teach you how to give them and supervise your taking them. A rare person does better on vitamin B12b (hydroxocobalamin) tablets, rather than injection.

Take hydroxocobalamin acetate tablets 500 mg, one to 20 tablets daily, first thing in the morning. One to 20 tablets sounds like strange directions. "Play" with the dosage to find out how much you need to feel your best. (Officially this is called a "therapeutic trial," an old and honored way to test.) If eight tablets work as well as 20, then stay with eight. You'll be pleased to learn that the tablets are small.

A few patients need the tablets several times a day. Some patients do best if they shoot the injectable B12b into an inch of water in a glass and drink it. One or two of my patients squirt the injectable B12b beneath their tongues and hold it there until some of it is absorbed.

Folic acid is a B vitamin. It's not a do-it-yourself vitamin. Those who take medication for epilepsy should work especially close with their physicians when taking folic acid. Everyone should have a blood test for folic acid. If you are low in folic acid, it's most important to take the vitamin. Never take folic acid unless you are either getting regular injections of vitamin B12b (hydroxocobalamin) or have regular blood tests to be certain your B12 level is normal. Best source: 1 mg tablet one to three times a day.

L-Carnitine (vitamin B-T) is moving up into the ranks of important vitamins. L-carnitine (*do not take* DL-carnitine or D-carnitine) helps fat metabolism. It's also important for energy production on the cellular level. It may prove especially important for people who are losing weight. Many people have noticeably more energy when taking it. Use L-carnitine capsules, 250 mg, one capsule daily. L-carnitine works best when taken on an empty stomach.

Because this vitamin has not yet been used in large amounts by great numbers of people, you should stay in touch with your physician while on it.

People often feel better and have more energy if they take a crude source of vitamins in addition to purified vitamins, that is, if they get their vitamins from foods, as they occur in nature. But many people are sensitive to crude vitamins. This is especially true of crude B vitamins. They may make you hungry and defeat your weight-loss program if they're incompatible with your chemistry. You cannot improve your health by taking vitamins—or anything else—which do not agree with your particular body chemistry.

Cautiously, try crude B vitamins and gradually build up to the desired level. I suggest, however, that you first settle down on your diet and vitamin program for several weeks.

Desiccated liver powder furnishes a crude source of B vitamins.

Although many people are allergic to it, more people can tolerate it than can tolerate the various forms of yeast. I take half a teaspoon of desiccated liver powder a day. Many patients can function well and feel good only if they take injections both of vitamin B12b and of crude liver.

If tolerated, it's a good idea to eat beef liver once a week. Most of my patients, however, find liver incompatible with their biochemistry.

Vitamin C is, of course, one of the big-name vitamins, and rightfully so, considering the body's critical need for it. *Best source*: vitamin C powder (ascorbic acid) is my first choice. I recommend taking ascorbic acid powder (vitamin C powder), very fine, a quarter teaspoon in a full glass of room-temperature water three times a day. Some people need much more. Check with your physician before taking larger amounts.

NOTE: You may mix all powders (such as vitamin C and dolomite) in the same water.

Forget about sterility, miscarriages and kidney stones caused by vitamin C. Those turned out to be old wives' tales told by the anti-vitamin establishment.

The vitamin C powder should be very fine, like flour, not coarse like sugar, and dissolved in water before you take it. You would think it made no difference whether it was fine or rough. I once telephoned the manufacturer and asked about the difference between the fine and the rough.

"To make it fine, we grind it more," was his remark.

Why people tolerate the fine better, I have no idea—but they do.

As an alternative, you can try ascorbic acid in a clear capsule of 500 mg. Take two capsules three times a day, or tablets. Tablets should state on the label, "Sugar and starch free."

Calcium ascorbate, sodium ascorbate, and timed-release capsules are available, but you should not take them without a physician's advice. I have one patient who is so allergic to all forms of vitamin C that she can only break an ampule of injectable vitamin c, shake it into water and drink it.

Pregnancy and Vitamins

If pregnant, stay under the close care of your physician and get his approval for taking any supplements. Be sure he has a current list of the supplements you take.

There is one caution about taking vitamin C (and all other vitamins) in large amounts while pregnant.

Either:

1. Gradually and drastically cut down the dosage beginning at the fifth month of pregnancy, or,

2. At the start of the fifth month, *inform the doctor who will be taking care of your infant* after it's born that you are on a large amount of vitamin C and other vitamins.

He probably won't know how to handle the situation. Inform him or her that:

If you decide not to nurse your infant, or if you try and fail to nurse your infant, the doctor must give the baby vitamin C (and other vitamins) and gradually cut down on the dose. Otherwise, the infant will be stressed if it goes from your high body supply of vitamin C (and other vitamins) to the poor supply of vitamins found in baby formulas.

If you nurse your infant, (and please do!) this will not be a problem.

Often doctors treat patients as if they are idiots. Doctors say, "Yes, yes," and pat them on the shoulder when they are not even listening. To get your doctors' attention and be sure he or she hears what you are saying, not only *tell* your doctor or doctors who will deliver you and care for your newborn infant, but send them registered letters with the information.

Vitamin E: Take as d-alpha tocopheryl *acetate* capsule of 200 units, one after breakfast or lunch (NOTE: *Tocopheryl* is sometimes spelled *tocopherol*.)

Warning: Vitamin E may cause excessive bleeding during surgery. Many surgeons advise that patients stop taking it 10 days before surgery. It helps protect against the type of blood clots that may come on following surgery. It is advisable to begin taking E again on the second day following surgery. Be sure to ask your surgeon's advice.

For the same reason, pregnant women should take no more than 100 units of vitamin E daily.

A few people out of a hundred develop high blood pressure when on more than 200 units of vitamin E a day. I very well remember one lady from Philadelphia. The 400 units of vitamin E she took each day caused her high blood pressure.

Unsaturated Oils

Unsaturated oils are as important as vitamins, but people often neglect them.

A fatty membrane surrounds each of the billions of cells in our bodies. We must furnish the cells with unsaturated fats to replace those lost by the membranes. All the food for maintenance, energy and reproduction must pass through the cell walls. All the vitamins, minerals, oxygen and the waste products of metabolism such as carbon dioxide, must go through the cell membrane. It's critically important that we keep these membranes intact and in good health.

Hormone-like fats with the catchy name *prostaglandins* are essential for our body chemistry. We must have unsaturated fats in our diets for our bodies to make prostaglandins. Prostaglandins are especially important for smooth muscle tissue, such as that found in the intestinal tract and in the uterus. Also, prostaglandins help lower blood-pressure.

An article in the scientific journal *Nature* stated that fish oils decrease blood clotting and increase bleeding time. The eating of oily fish may explain the low rate of heart disease in Greenland and among the Eskimos. Cod liver oil is a fish oil.

For good health, we need both types of fats, saturated and unsaturated. Saturated fats come mostly from meats.

Unsaturated fats help the body handle saturated fats and lower cholesterol levels. Most vegetable oils—except olive oil—contain generous quantities of unsaturated fats. Avoid peanut oil, corn oil and margarine.

Warning: If you overheat or burn them, all oils and fats turn toxic and carcinogenic.

Since various oils contain various combinations of essential unsaturated fats, I recommend that people take both cod liver oil and linseed oil. Buy linseed oil at a health food store. *Do not* take linseed oil bought at a paint or hardware store! The label on the linseed oil, now often called flaxseed oil, must read: "cold-pressed, no preservatives." I suggest one teaspoon every day—no more.

Oils used in cooking don't count. Heat destroys some of the helpful properties. After opening oils, keep them refrigerated.

Minerals

Calcium and **magnesium** must always be present in the body in about a two-to-one ratio. Advertisements that push calcium without also pushing magnesium are doing everyone a great disservice. If you take calcium alone, you may actually reduce your body's calcium level. We live in a society that is dangerously lacking in magnesium.

Take one calcium carbonate tablet (600 mg) two times a day, plus one magnesium oxide tablet (250 mg) two or three times a day. As an alternative, try dolomite powder—half teaspoon in water twice daily. Note: Some dolomite has been found to contain toxic amounts of heavy metals. Check out the dolomite you plan to take with the company that distributes it. Get a letter from them listing the heavy metals it contains.

Some people claim the dolomite is insoluble and therefore cannot be used by the body as a source of calcium and magnesium. Nonsense. I know that it can be used because I see the clinical results that come from using it.

I take dolomite.

As a rough test of your calcium level, snap the end of your fingernails. If the nails are soft and weak, you probably need more calcium.

Exercise is a vital part of the calcium-magnesium prescription. You can follow a super perfect diet, but if you don't walk, you will not be able to retain calcium in your bones and will develop osteoporosis. Walk for at least an hour and five minutes daily all at one time, preferably in the daylight. If you can't walk, crawl!

If pregnant or nursing a baby, be sure to ask your doctor about your increased mineral needs.

Take **selenium** in a 200 *mcg* tablet. Only take tablets labeled "kelp-free, yeast-free." Take one tablet daily in the evening. Selenium helps prevent cancer and is an antioxidant.

Zinc gluconate—take one 60 mg capsule three times a day. This is very important to prevent infections and to help prevent cancer.

Micro-minerals

Kelp—one tablet every other day—is an excellent source of trace or microminerals. Because kelp contains iodine, it may cause acne skin lesions in those who are susceptible. If that happens, stop taking it and depend upon yeast or vegetables for your trace minerals.

The world of vitamin-taking is wide and deep. Finding your absolute best level of various vitamins and other supplements can take a lifetime. Study my book *Mega-Nutrients*.

7

The Simplified Newbold Diet

Fat people age early and therefore die early.

— ARISTOTLE

PAGLIACCI: LAUGHTER THROUGH TEARS

Thelma, the wife of a famous comic we'll call Don Sordi, visited my office before her husband's appointment to tell me about his troubles. Tragedy, street-wisdom and determination showed in her garishly-painted mid-forties face.

"Don has high blood pressure," she told me. "Last month he had a minor stroke. The doctor gave him a 1200 calorie diet and told him to lose weight or else. He tried to follow the diet, but like every other one he's tried, he felt horrible on it and couldn't stick to it.

"His career is about to blow away. In six weeks he's doing a *live* TV special. The doctor's afraid the stress will make Don have another stroke. He's turned morbid. He's convinced they're doing the show live so everybody can watch him die on stage."

"How much does he weigh?" I asked.

"Nobody knows. He refuses to get on the scales. But take my word for it, Don's fat. He must weigh three tons. He eats enough to feed a herd of elephants. I've read your books and I'm sure you're the only doctor who can help him." After a pause, she added, "I forgot to mention that he hates doctors and loathes diets."

"Any medical trouble other than high blood pressure?"

Don's medical history was a roll call of the degenerative ills that come from living in what politicians tell us is "the greatest civilization the world has ever known." Don suffered not only from obesity, but from many of the complications that go with it: high blood pressure, borderline diabetes, arthritic pains in his left knee and spastic colon. Half the time he lived in a black hole of depression.

"Is he too far gone for help? Do you want to hear more?"

"He sounds like my typical patient. Tell me the rest of it."

Don despised all restrictions from buttoned shirt collars to keeping receipts for his accountant. Women had once been his first passion. Food came second. Now, at age 52, he still perused the ladies, but food had become more important.

While working the nightclub circuit in the early days, Don would breeze into a hotel in a new city and palm a $200 tip on the bell captain and tell him to send a few gals to his suite for a three A.M. party.

After his last show, while still warmed and reassured by the applause echoing through his heart, Don would lock the door to his dressing room and nibble on sugar-sprinkled wafers while quaffing splits of champagne.

"Now you get to see the real show!" he would announce to the girls after returning to his hotel following his last performance.

Don would do a soft-shoe dance and throw the girls one-liners raw enough to make Hugh Hefner blush. Later, he'd indulge in more champagne while eating three-inch-thick caviar sandwiches. For dessert, he worked through a tall stack of ice-cream topped *crepes suzette*.

"Don't forget, the party ain't over till the fat man throws up," he would shout as he belly-laughed and applauded.

How did his wife know about all this?

She had been one of the girls in Kansas City. Instead of leaving, she had stayed to help after he threw up, after he staggered to bed, after he got the shakes and wept from loneliness and fear that when he went on stage tomorrow night he might not be funny.

"You want to know why I'm still with him?" Thelma said. "I don't have the heart to walk out on him. Without me, he would fall apart." She gave an ironic smile. "Besides, I'm too old to go back to working the hotels. Don's failed on every imaginable diet. Do you think you can help him?"

"Look," I told Thelma, "people think that because I'm a well-known doctor, they only need to visit me a time or two and bask in my aura. Whether I can help him depends on his cooperation. Vitamins alone won't solve his problems. If he won't eat the foods that are compatible with his biochemistry and stay away from things in the environment that knock out his appetite center, nothing will help him."

"I'll do my best to see that he cooperates."

"It will take time and work, but if he'll follow my suggestions, I can show him how to completely turn his life around."

"How long will it take?"

"He should stay here in New York for two weeks. I can teach him how to test foods for incompatibilities and help him through the withdrawal stage. After we have him going in the right direction, he'll lose two to three pounds a week. He'll still need supervision. We can give him telephone appointments. He should come back to New York in about six to eight weeks and stay for a day or two."

"He won't stay two weeks. Just write down what your diet is and I'll put him on it."

"It's too complicated to do that way. It won't work."

"Just write some notes for me. Let's give it a try."

Like the King of Siam who owned and commanded all that surrounded him, the next day Don made his grand entrance into my office, along with his entourage: his wife, his "social secretary," and his two bodyguards. I wondered why he hadn't brought along his chauffeur, his chef and the two "nurses" that slept in the room next to him in case he had "breathing difficulties" during the night.

Surprisingly, Don's round face was pale. I had expected the telltale red face of hypertension. As I looked closer, I realized that he had hidden his true skin color behind pancake makeup and powder.

Pale pink, his silk suit was cut so large and flowing he could have shared it with a twin brother. The fragrant gardenia in the lapel matched his worn-open-at-the-neck white silk shirt. Were his Gucci loafers supposed to remind the world that he had money?

"Well, here we are, the King of Comedy with his court jesters. Would it have been cheaper by the dozen?" Don quipped.

He should also have brought along his gag writers.

I showed Don and his wife into my private office. Not wanting to embarrass himself by trying to fit into a chair, Don chose the couch. He perched on the edge as if not planning to stay very long.

Don fidgeted while I took a medical history.

"How much alcohol do you use?" I asked.

"A little now and then."

"Winston Churchill thought a bottle of brandy a day was only a little now and then."

"So, I drink. What else do you want to know?"

Typical of self-made, successful men, Don saw himself above the laws of man and nature. Such people admit to no weaknesses and will bow neither to kings nor gods. Often they would rather die than let anyone see their weaknesses, especially another man, especially a man who is himself successful.

"Were you breast fed or bottle fed?"

"What the hell kind of question is that?"

"Most patients I see with medical problems and weight problems like yours were bottle fed."

"I was bottle fed," he said and sulked.

As expected, he also had a family history of diabetes.

While I questioned him for three more minutes, Don's restlessness all but made him jump out the window.

"I'm not allowed to smoke in here? What kind of office is it where you can't smoke?"

"From what your wife told me, you have several serious medical problems. I'm trying to help."

"Stop the merry-go-round and let me off. There's nothing wrong with me. I thought I was here to pick up a handful of vitamins."

"What I do is more complicated than that. I need for you to stay here in New York for at least two weeks so I can help you get started on a weight loss program."

"That's impossible! Not even two days. I have to get back to the coast."

"Your public loves you, but Mother Nature doesn't. She only wants to use you to push up daisies."

"Doc, one thing I gotta say for you: You got one hell of a bedside manner."

"If you want a Hollywood doctor who'll pat your hand and baby you, you've got the wrong doctor."

"Okay, you leveled with me. Now I'm going to level with you."

"Pray do."

"And a comic," he said to his wife. " 'Pray do,' this guy's a comic!"

"You said you were going to level with me."

"Okay, I'm leveling with you. I can't sit here any longer without a cigarette. Even with a cigarette I couldn't sit here any longer. I got to move it, cruise around some. Why don't you get in the stretch with us and finish telling me what to do while we float back to the Sherry?"

I had two more patients to see during the afternoon, but perhaps I should give Don priority. He was courting death. Like Mount Rushmore, Don was a national treasure. He did more than make people forget their troubles. Last year he raised $20 million for charities.

I handed his wife a sheet of information for new patients, a lab order sheet and a physical examination form.

Don plucked a cigarette from a gold-lined case pavéed with diamonds.

The white Mercedes stretch limousine waiting at the curb in front of my office looked long enough to transport the fifth and sixth armies, but felt crowded when all of us settled inside. A guard closed the door. The two giant white German shepherd dogs that insisted upon putting their paws in my lap and licking my face made me feel even more crowded.

"Okay, now tell me what I'm supposed to eat."

"The cigarette smoke and the perfumed dogs are too much for me. Let me out. I'll get a taxi. If your secretary will come with me, I'll give her some notes about your diet. I'll go over them with you at the hotel."

That year, March was a lion. In the cold wind and swirling snow I held my hand up to signal for a taxi.

The shy little brunette in her early twenties had long black lashes and big black eyes. They called the secretary "Tuesday." I discovered that Tuesday had nothing to write with and nothing to write on. After stopping at a stationery store, I discovered that she could neither take shorthand nor spell. Also, she confessed, she didn't type.

"I suppose nobody's perfect," I observed.

"You needn't be so cavalier about it."

"What does 'cavalier' have to do with it?"

"I'll explain sometime."

I later learned that Tuesday had heard the word cavalier on a TV game show. She had adopted the word and used it whenever she wanted to either impress someone or counter an argument.

Simplified Newbold Diet

I spoke the words as I wrote them on the first page of the tablet. "Simply speaking, the Newbold Diet takes patients off the new agricultural foods that have been added to mankind's diet during the past 5,000 to 10,000 years.

"In their place, the person who wants to lose weight eats mankind's traditional foods: meats, fish, fowl and small amounts of vegetables and perhaps some fruits.

"Drink nothing except water, at least one and a half quarts daily.

"Because people can be sensitive to certain foods and because those foods can knock out the appetite control center and send people on eating sprees, it's important to test each food by eating them one at a time.

"Also, environmental insults can knock out the appetite center—the appestat—and send people on eating sprees. Some people won't lose weight until they get away from common chemicals like those blown into the air by copy machines and laser printers. Incompatibility with flowers, perfume, tobacco smoke, carpeting, pets, etcetera, can make many people hungry."

"Come on!" Tuesday interrupted. "Don's not going to pay any attention to all those fancy words. He'll want you to tell him exactly what to eat, one, two, three."

Here's the simplified version of the Newbold Diet, one, two, three, that I gave her:

Step One: At each meal eat all of the *fresh* chicken*, fish*, veal, beef rib steak, porterhouse steak, lamb, pork, desired or other fresh meats desired. Include some of the fat. Eat none of the burned or browned fat or meat. Cook with electricity. If they are compatible with his chemistry, he should get most of his calories from beef rib steaks.

Step Two: It's not required, but if he wants it, he may have half a cup of a *fresh, raw* vegetable three times a day *with* his meal—if he can find vegetables that are compatible with his chemistry. No root vegetables such as carrots, parsnips and potatoes.

*See notes on fish and chicken, pages 71 and 72.

Step Three: It's not required, but if he wants it, he may have one cup of *fresh, raw, compatible* fruit three times a day *after* his meals. Many people are unable to eat any fruits and lost weight.

Step Four: Drink nothing but plain bottled spring water, at least one and a half quarts a day.

Step Five: Test foods one at a time to learn which ones make him feel bad or send him on an eating spree.

Step Six: Avoid environmental insults like copy machine odors, flowers, perfume, smoke from tobacco, carpeting, pets, etcetera.

Step Seven: Walk outdoors one hour a day, preferably during the daylight hours. If he can't walk for an hour, he should do his best and gradually work up to an hour.

"Do you really think Don's going to get rid of his flowers and his dogs and eat like that?" Tuesday asked.

"To be honest with you, I don't think he will. He's in too big a hurry. He needs much more help and information. I need to teach him how to test meats and other foods so he can learn exactly which foods his body chemistry can handle. He'll need help with withdrawal symptoms and a dozen other problems that will come up."

"When Don sees this diet, he'll have his bodyguards toss you down the back stairs."

Don's hotel suite looked and smelled like a florist shop. When Thelma joined me to read over the diet, I told her that the flowers and the perfumed dogs (even unperfumed dogs) could knock out the *turn-off* cells in Don's appestat and make him spree eat.

"Flowers can make people fat!" she said.

"Yes, flowers can make some people fat."

She looked at me as if I were Dr. No from outer space.

In the next room I heard sounds from a Laurel and Hardy movie. Don had to leave my office and rush back to his hotel to watch a Laurel and Hardy movie!

"Is this diet a joke?" Thelma asked after reading it. "You're going to let him eat all that meat and cholesterol?"

"If he wants a high fat diet and leaves off all grains, milk and milk products, nuts and table sugar *his cholesterol level will fall*, or his high density lipoprotein will rise, which is equivalent to having the cholesterol fall. I've researched the subject and published several papers about it in medical journals.

"Recently I learned that two generations ago DuBois at Cornell and McCallum at Johns Hopkins observed the same thing and wrote about it in the *American Journal of Biological Chemistry.*

"The *Journal of the American Medical Association* published a cholesterol study of over 4000 people in the town of Tecumseh, Michigan. (See "Independence of Serum Lipid Levels and Dietary Habits: The Tecumseh Study," 1976.) What people ate had no influence on their cholesterol levels. *Weight was the only factor that influenced the cholesterol levels. If people were overweight, their cholesterol levels were high.*

"An article in this week's *Journal of the American Medical Association* said that two-thirds of the people could eat whatever they wanted. Food has no effect on their cholesterol levels. The article intimated that the advertising by food manufacturers had unnecessarily frightened the American public about cholesterol.

"I'll have some more information about cholesterol typed up and mailed to you. Forget about cholesterol for the moment. Losing weight is the best thing he can do to lower his cholesterol."

"What about the impurities in meat?"

"They're no worse than the impurities in wheat. The wheat that goes into breakfast cereals has been chemically sprayed to kill insects, sprayed again to kill mold and sprayed to keep out rats. Even so, it's full of dead insect heads and legs. The USDA allows two rat droppings per quart of wheat. I'll send up some more information about impurities in wheat.

"Everything in life is a compromise, including food. Mother's milk is radioactive and contains PCBs, still, it's the best compromise for babies. The question is, which food is the best compromise for Don's particular body chemistry."

"What about cancer?"

"Fats are not cancer-producing if certain precautions are taken. I'll also mail you some information about the relationship between meat, fat and cancer."

"You're sure it's all right to go on a diet like this?"

"He should first have a physical examination and the laboratory tests I ordered. After I get the results, he should be able to start the diet."

Not So Simple

"Losing weight and keeping it off is more complicated than you realize. Don still doesn't have nearly enough information to do it on his own. Some of the foods won't agree with him. I need to teach him how to test foods."

"I'm sure we'll manage with what you've given us."

"I haven't had time to list the vitamin and other supplements he needs."

"Don has vitamins."

Little did they know the complexity of the subject. They were babes in the woods.

"I haven't explained withdrawal reactions. When he changes his diet, he'll feel much worse for three or four days. He can feel very ill from withdrawal symptoms."

That was it. I was being dismissed. Tuesday had been right. This was Don's way of throwing me down the backstairs.

My last words were, "Don't forget, he has to stop drinking; otherwise, he won't lose weight. . . ."

It was a pity, but Don was going to fail—all that useless suffering! Failures always make me feel sad.

8

The More Sophisticated Newbold Diet

Each patient carries his own doctor inside him. We are at our best when we give the doctor who resides within a chance to work.

—ALBERT SCHWEITZER

DON REVISITED

Two weeks later another scattering of snow whirled down between the New York skyscrapers as I took Tuesday's telephone call.

"Don's doctor got him off booze."

"That's important. It must have been rough."

"He almost went into D.T.s. He needed nurses around the clock to give him vitamin shots and something to relax him."

"Is he better?"

"For a few days he was better. Then he started on your diet and went crazy and started eating 10 times more sweets than ever. Now he's in the pits. Thelma wants you to come out and try to do something."

"Are they ready to listen to me?"

"Don says he'll do anything."

A smiling Tuesday met me as I entered the air terminal in Palm Springs. The chauffeur took my bag and led us outside to another white Mercedes limousine. The sun shone and the green palm fronds moved in the breeze. The people wore informal clothes and smiled relaxedly.

"Don's spread is in a town called Rancho Mirage," Tuesday explained. "It's south of Palm Springs. More exclusive."

After we had driven a few minutes, I saw little evidence of a town, but much evidence of the local citizen-heroes: Dinah Shore Drive, Frank Sinatra Drive, Bob Hope Drive. I wondered if the town had any book shops. We passed expensive houses and estates.

At last the limo paused as two guards opened massive Florentine iron gates and waved us through. Eventually, the blacktop meandered to a parking lot near a garage that could easily hold a dozen cars. Two pumps for gasoline stood at the far end of the lot.

Slate-topped paths curved past two swimming pools and restful buildings made of white-washed brick topped with roofs of dull red tiles. Only the relaxing sound of water flowing from fountains broke the peace. Combining green grass, flowering bushes and palm trees, a landscape artist had made the ground look as if nature had spent a thousand years weaving everything together. How many jokes had it cost to build such magnificence?

After leading me to one of several guest houses, Tuesday said Don would see me soon.

An hour later, Tuesday ushered me into the semi-dark master bedroom. Like the hotel room in New York, flowers crowded the oversized room. Don's two perfumed white German shepherd dogs resting across the foot of his Czar-sized bed lifted their heads and looked at me.

In New York I had seen Don at his best, wearing makeup, wearing his pink silk suit and Gucci loafers. Now his face could belong to a Bowery bum on Monday morning. Circles of liver-colored bags surrounded his eyes and sagged down to his cheekbones. When he saw me, he switched off the TV as if ashamed to be caught watching a soap. He looked down at the satin spread across his lap and picked at it.

"So, give me a funny line," he muttered.

"You're at the end of the road," I said. "No laughs here. Nothing but a hard place."

"So shoot me. Bang! Bang!"

"Sometimes people need to hit their head on the rock at the end of the road before they're ready to listen."

"My regular doctor says that if I don't lose weight and get my blood pressure down, I won't be able to do the TV gig. Once I had pneumonia when I went on stage in Detroit, but I didn't feel this bad.

If I can't make it, that pushy William Morris Agency will get someone else to do my show. Believe me, you got my attention."

"Good."

"Your diet is one bitch on roller skates."

"Only the first three days."

Thelma joined us.

"What happened?" I asked her.

"You said Don had to stop drinking before he could lose weight. His doctor got him dry. It wasn't easy. After he was off the booze, Don started your diet. On the second day he felt so tense and depressed he nearly flipped. He went on an eating spree, then started the diet again. Now he feels lousy again. What's wrong?"

I explained that Don had both a *Type-A* (spree) and a *Type-B* (addiction) weight problem. At the moment it was the *Type-B* problem that was laying him low. *He was suffering from withdrawal symptoms.*

The Food-Mood Connection

"Don has food addictions," I told Thelma. "He keeps eating foods to avoid withdrawal reactions like the one he's having now. The foods keep him overweight. When he goes on my diet, he stops eating the addictive foods and he has withdrawal symptoms.

"When you were in New York I warned you about withdrawal symptoms. I don't know why people never hear me when I tell them about the withdrawal awfuls. Maybe the word 'withdrawal' doesn't mean anything to them."

"I didn't know withdrawal could be this bad."

"You don't realize that food is a strong force. You were too cocky about the diet. For someone as addicted as Don, the diet can be complicated. You need help. I keep telling people—but they never hear me— withdrawing from a food that's addictive for you is no different from withdrawing from heroin. He'll feel like this for three or four days."

"So what does he do for three or four days?" Thelma asked.

"He could go back on a regular diet, then change to my diet slowly. But that would take much more time. He's in a hurry and I can't stay out here forever. He's this far along. I think he should sweat it out and get past the withdrawal stage all at once."

"What happens if he sticks to it?"

"He'll feel bad for a few days. Two Bufferins four times a day will help. Valium would help, but then Valium would be a problem. He would become addicted to Valium. Then he would feel this way again when he came off Valium."

For three days Tuesday and I sat around the pool and sunned ourselves while Don suffered. I learned that Tuesday was a would-be actress. They called her Tuesday because she spent Tuesday nights with Don.

Then, as predicted, on the third day, Don felt much better.

During the middle of the fourth night, Thelma caught him raiding the kitchen for cookies and champagne. It happened again on the fifth night.

Thelma attacked me as if it were my fault.

"We're missing something," I told Thelma. "Don has a *Type-A* weight problem in addition to his *Type-B* weight problem."

"Type A, type Z, who gives a damn. What do we do?"

"Something knocks out his appestat. That's the appetite control center in the brain. It's one of three things: Something he's eating. Something in his water. Or something in his environment."

"So what do we *do*?"

"Let's assume it's something in his room. We'll strip a spare bedroom and move him in there."

We stripped a room: removed the carpeting and draperies and the furniture and left only a mattress. No flowers. No dogs. No scented products. All-cotton sheets. All-cotton pillow. All-cotton pajamas.

Furthermore, we kept all chemicals out of the room: no insect sprays, no wax or polish. Much to the maid's displeasure, I had her use white vinegar to clean the windows and mirrors and clean the bathroom by scrubbing it with baking soda.

Don, and everyone who entered the room, stopped using all scented products. He used baking soda to brush his teeth and as mouthwash.

When Don saw the room, he said *"Sieg heil!"* and gave me a *"Sieg heil"* salute.

"Any of the things we took out could knock out your appestat and send you on an eating spree. We could have taken out one item at a time. We could take the flowers out this week, then remove the dogs next week, then the carpet. . . . But that way we might all die of old age before we found out what's hitting your appestat."

He started calling me Dr. S. H.

We must have hit it right. Once we stripped the bedroom, he stopped spree eating.

Test Beef First

We began testing foods one at a time to learn wehther any of them would give him an unpleasant reaction or send him on an eating spree.

"Why test fish-fowl-meats first?" Thelma asked.

"We need to find a few high calorie 'old foods' that can become the backbone of his diet. If we tested celery and found that it was compatible with his biochemistry, it wouldn't help much. He would starve to death if celery made up the main part of his diet. Once we find some fish-fowl-meat that he tolerates, he can eat those while we test fruits and vegetables around them. It's simple. You'll see. Beef rib steak is the high calorie 'old food' that's usually well tolerated, so let's start by testing it."

The chauffeur drove Tuesday and me into town. We bought a pink, unaged, mid-rib beef steak. I had the butcher cut it one-and-one-quarter-inch thick and leave all the fat on it. Because most people feel tired and toxic after eating the deckle, I had him remove the deckle, which is a thick section of meat just beyond the rib and is often sold with the rib.

The Chinese cook looked as if he were about to attack me with a cleaver as I stood by and watched him boil the steak in bottled spring water. I had the cook keep cutting into the steak to be certain it remained pink in the center. (We later tested meats *broiled* with electricity.)

On the test day, Don ate nothing for at least two hours before the test meal. I cut off one-eighth of an inch of meat and fat around the edge of the steak. That removed meat and fat that had been exposed to the air and become oxidized.

Don then ate half of the steak. At my direction, he ate a small amount of the white fat along with the lean meat. There was no seasoning on the steak. He was allowed to drink water with it. He ate nothing for at least two hours after eating the steak.

He had no reaction from eating the rib steak. Because he had no significant reaction (like hunger, headache, pain in joints, gas, etc.) from the rib steak, the next day we repeated the test on rib steak. We then moved on to test porterhouse steak and chuck steak.

Some people who consult me find beef unsuited for their biochemistry. I have a Jewish patient in Staten Island who can only tolerate pork. In my experience treating thousands of patients, however, I have found mid-rib beef rib steaks the most commonly tolerated food. The second-best tolerated: porterhouse steak.

"How do I find out whether my chemistry is compatible with beef—or with fish or chicken?" you ask.

You test. When testing remember you might react differently to meats from different origins. Some people can eat IBP (a midwestern beef), but not beef grown in New Jersey and vice versa. Some people can eat cryovaced meat, and others must have hung meat. Ask your butcher where the meat came from and whether it was wrapped in plastic and chilled (cryovaced) or hung in a refrigerated truck and shipped to your location.

This beef thing can be complicated. My butcher, for example, without telling me, started buying his meat in a different part of the country. I was tired and depressed for half a week before I found out what was causing the trouble.

Another point: Always have your meat cut fresh. Never buy it from the bins where it lies wrapped in plastic. That is important.

Many people think meat doesn't agree with them when they are merely buying meat grown in the wrong part of the country, or meat that is aged, or is too young, has been cut and lying in plastic, or has been cooked with gas, or they have been eating browned or burned fat.

Testing Other Meats

After finishing your beef tests, if you wish, try veal, lamb, and pork. Be sure to cook the pork well. Test only meats that have a generous amount of fat. For example, lean thin-cut veal is of no value. You'll only become ill if you eat significant amounts of it.

How do I know? I've used this diet on thousands of patients for more than 20 years. I didn't collect my information from other people's books and papers. I learned from my own reactions and those of my patients.

Fish

The first problem with fish is, as a rule, people are less likely to tolerate fish than red meats.

Second problem with fish: People often do not get enough to eat when eating fish. If left hungry, people are more likely to cheat on their diets.

Third problem: Fish are our most dangerously contaminated food. As a rule, I ask people not to eat fish more than once a week. If you plan on eating fish more than once a week, you should make arrangements for your local health department to analyze the fish you eat for chemicals and heavy metals. Repeat the analysis every two months.

Test fresh fish. Test oily fish because they will satisfy you better. Test fish such as blue fish, black fish, salmon, shark, halibut and mackerel. Steam or boil the fish. Be certain to use spring water, not chlorinated tap water.

Then, if you wish, test shellfish such as shrimp, scallops and oysters. Because they contain little fat, they will fail to satisfy you and for this reason should not be eaten frequently.

Do not eat raw oysters or other raw shellfish. We've had too many epidemics of hepatitis traced back to shellfish.

Some of my patients make a meal of red meat and for a change of pace have fish as a side dish.

If your test shows that you tolerate shellfish, you might want to put shrimp or some other shellfish on your steak now and then for flavoring.

Fowl

Most of my patients do not do well on fowl. Personally, I've never found any fowl that does not leave me feeling tired and toxic.

The best tolerated types are range-fed fowl. You may tolerate one brand and not another. I have two patients who can tolerate no commercial chicken, but can tolerate the chickens they grow on their own farms.

Test the light meat and the dark meat separately. You may tolerate one and not the other. Most people tolerate dark meat best.

Follow the same directions given for testing red meat. If you wish, test chicken and other fowl such as rock cornish hen, turkey, duck and goose. You should make a point of eating the skin of fowl. It contains a high percentage of the bird's fat.

Some of my patients make meals of red meat and eat cold fowl for lunch or for snacks.

Butter

Butter is the only dairy product which I found commonly tolerated. Use sweet, unsalted butter. If you react to butter, then clarify it and test again. Some people can tolerate only clarified butter.

(To clarify butter, place butter in the top of a double boiler. Put water in the bottom of the boiler. Heat until the butter melts. Skim off the part of the butter that floats and throw it away. The clear middle layer is the clarified butter. Save that and refrigerate it. Throw away the residual butter that covers the bottom of the pan.)

Butter can be the dieter's friend. If you get a steak with too little fat on it—as you will in many countries other than the United States and Argentina—you can add butter to improve the fat content.

At this point some people will scream about cholesterol and the heavy calorie content of butter. See Chapter 17 on cholesterol.

I must admit that I haven't done control studies to find out what happens to cholesterol levels when butter is eaten on a grain–milk–sugar-free diet.

I have the clinical impression that people should limit the amount of butter they eat.

Do not eat margarine. We don't know enough about its biological effects.

As mentioned, fats have more than twice as many calories as carbohydrates. The secret is that fats satisfy four or five times as much as carbohydrates. For that reason you lose weight while eating fats if you leave out carbohydrates.

Vegetables

Fish-fowl-meats make up the backbone of your diet. That's why we test them first. Fruits and vegetables are only play foods. They may furnish bioflavonoids, micro-minerals and possibly other unknown factors.

Once we work out which fish-fowl-meats you can tolerate, then, if you wish, you may test vegetables and fruits.

To test, eat only one vegetable at a time (eat it along with a meat that you've tested and cleared). Do not repeat the vegetable for 72 hours. Have no more than half a cup. For example, if you have celery for lunch, allow three days to pass before eating celery again.

Once you have cleared the vegetable—that is, you have discovered that it does not make you hungry and does not give you any side reactions such as gas—then you may have half a cup of a fresh raw vegetable with each meal, but no more than three times a day. (No potatoes, carrots or other root vegetables such as turnips or parsley. No beans or peas.)

Eat vegetables only with your meat. Do not eat them as snacks. Leave off those that disagree with you. Peel vegetables wherever possible. If unable to peel a vegetable (such as spinach), wash and rinse very well before eating.

Fruits

It's not required, but if you wish you may have one cup of *fresh, raw* fruit three times a day *after* your meal. (No bananas, grapes, oranges, mangos or pineapple.)

But first test and clear each fruit. Eat only one fruit at a time and do not repeat it for 72 hours. If you have peaches for lunch, for example, allow three days to pass before eating peaches again. Even when testing fruit, eat it only *after* eating one of your tested and cleared meats. Do not eat fruit as a snack.

Peel fruits wherever possible. If unable to peel a fruit (such as berries), wash and rinse well before eating.

Some fruits will prove incompatible. They'll give you gas or make you tired, hungry, or give you some other symptom. Such fruits should be avoided. Rotate among the fruits that agree with you.

Most dieters should not eat *any* fruit. The other night after dinner I had a nice ripe cantaloupe. The next morning I had trouble concentrating and for two days I felt hungry. *Never eat dried fruit.*

If you fail to lose two to three pounds a week, cut back on your fruit. Try having it twice a day. If you are not losing the correct amount of weight, reduce it to once a day. A few people must leave off fruit altogether to lose satisfactorily.

Remember, fruits may make you hungry. If so, leave off all fruits.

Water and Other Beverages

Water can make you hungry if you are sensitive to it and it knocks out your appestat. Test waters by drinking one water for two days, then switch to another water for two days, etc. Observe whether you feel better on one water than another. If you aren't sure, repeat the testing cycle several times.

Two hundred known chemicals—some radioactive—contaminate New York's drinking water. Yet New York has one of the best drinking waters in the country. Florida has the worst water I've come across. The chlorine in some of the water in that state is strong enough to bleach your kidneys.

Bottled spring water may be great—or terrible. Some of the companies use plastic bottles that leach chemicals into the water. Water may be shipped in tank cars before it's bottled. After being emptied, tank cars may be sterilized with chemicals that contaminate the next shipment of water.

Bacterial counts are too high in some spring waters.

Other waters, for no understandable reason, cause reactions in some people. I have a patient who had to test 75 waters before finding a water wholly compatible with her chemistry. One of my patients moved to Hawaii because that was the only place she could tolerate the water.

At the moment, the best tolerated waters in New York are Poland Spring and Deerpark. Next year that may not be true.

I filter my water through charcoal, then distill it with a stainless steel distiller and store it in the refrigerator in glass bottles.

Simply boiling tap water for 10 minutes drives out many chemicals and greatly reduces the chlorine content. Boiling, however, concentrates the fluoride, so don't boil it for more than 10 minutes. If you fill your bottle with boiled water only halfway and shake it, you'll get oxygen back into it and the water will taste better.

On this diet, *you will be sick unless you drink at least one and a half quarts of water daily. Do not drink commercially distilled water or filtered water.* It's a good idea to drink one brand of bottled water exclusively. Later switch to another water for two days, then go to another and another to discover which brand suits you best. You want the water that is the most compatible with your chemistry, not necessarily the water that tastes best. It always amazes people when they learn they can react unfavorably to water.

Until you reach normal weight, you should drink nothing but water. Especially you should not drink alcoholic beverages of any kind, herb teas, ordinary tea, coffee, decaffeinated coffee, diet soda or juices. All of these are likely to give you trouble by making you hungry or giving you some other sort of reaction.

"Why not drink black coffee or tea with lemon?" you ask. These have no calories, but many people have biochemistries that are incompatible with coffee or tea. They often knock out the *turn-off* cells in the appestat and make people hungry.

Diet colas in particular often strike the appestat and make people hungry. In a recent study cited by the American Cancer Society, people who drank diet sodas gained weight rather than lost weight. *Never drink diet sodas.* Don't trust ads. Smart men (the great hunters, the modern-day saber-toothed tigers of the Wall Street jungle) are trying to move food (money) from your cave into theirs. Like their cousins of yore, they will not hesitate to kill you to speed the transfer.

Starting Your Diet: Withdrawal Symptoms

Editors complain that in books I sometimes repeat myself. I do so because life has taught me that we forget at least half of what we read or hear.

When you change your diet, you will have withdrawal symptoms. You will feel ill for about four days, sometimes up to six days. Coming off foods like wheat and sugar is much like coming off heroin. During withdrawal, you can have any symptom you can name. Symptoms vary all the way from tiredness to flu-like blahs, to backache, abdominal pains, diarrhea and vomiting.

"Doctor Newbold, I don't feel good. I don't think your diet's agreeing with me."

Too often I get a call like that from a patient after following the diet plan for a couple of days. People often fail to hear me when I tell them to expect withdrawal symptoms.

If you change your diet gradually, your withdrawal symptoms will be milder, but will last longer. Some people do best to change all at once, and others do best to change slowly.

Modern Foods To Avoid

These new foods are likely to cause *Type-A* and *Type-B* weight problems:

1. **Grains** including wheat, rye, corn, rice and others. Also foods that contain grains such as spaghetti, pizza, bread, cake and breakfast cereal.
2. **Sugar**, as found on the table and in cakes, cookies, ice cream and soft drinks, and even in unsuspected items like salt, ketchup and canned peas.
3. **Milk** and milk products. These are in bread, cheese, ice cream, milk and yogurt. (Exception: Most people tolerate unsalted butter. It's more like beef fat than milk.)
4. **Nuts** are not a new food. Our European ancestors, however, had no nuts during the 65,000-year Würm glaciation. Perhaps that was long enough for many of my patients to have inherited a biochemistry that cannot function properly with nuts. Peanuts are the most poorly tolerated, though they are really a bean rather than a nut.
5. **Beans**.
6. **Peas**.
7. All **processed foods** such as frozen foods, dried foods, canned foods.
8. All **foods that must be cooked** before they can be eaten.

Sorry if these directions are beginning to sound a bit rigid. Try to remember that *these are not my directions. I'm only trying to tell you about Mother Nature's laws so you can obey them or not as you choose.*

At first, while still in the withdrawal phase, you'll look at the fish, fowl or meat on your plate and say, "No way!" But most of our calories must come from fish, fowl and meats. You—and I—must eat one of these foods at every meal or go hungry. Then you'll blame the food.

You're probably in the midst of withdrawal symptoms. During withdrawal, you want carbohydrates rather than meats. If you don't want the food, simply don't eat. After not eating for a few days, the food will become more appetizing.

"I never did like fish, fowl and meats," you say. Of course you didn't. That's one of the reasons you're overweight.

You'll be happy to learn that with time your tastes will change. Did you ever break up with a boy or girlfriend, run into them a year or two later and wonder what you ever saw in them? It will be the same after you go a few months without cake and ice cream.

Play a game. Pretend you're living 30,000 years ago. Make believe there's nothing other than fish-fowl-meat-limited raw vegetable-limited raw fruit to eat.

Eat Fats and Lose Weight

Forgive me, but I must repeat this important information. "Authorities" often advise weight losers to avoid fats. They've always heard that fats— gram for gram—have more than two times as many calories as lean meat or carbohydrates.

True, fats do have more than twice as many calories as carbohydrates and lean meats. Fats, however, satisfy us four or five times as much. For that reason, people who eat plenty of fats lose weight—*if* they go very light on the carbohydrates.

While on the Newbold Diet, *if you do not eat some of the fat you will become ill. You'll develop constipation or diarrhea and in general not feel well.* Again, let me remind you: *Do not eat the burned or browned fat.* Eat some of the white fat along with some of the lean meat. It takes time to learn the right amount of fat you need to eat.

In Summary

We isolated and tested one food at a time. I first test mid-rib beef steaks, then other meats. (No seasoning on test foods.)

Except for the test meal, eat your usual diet. At the test meal, have nothing to eat for two hours, then eat the test meal. Water is allowed with the test meal.

Have nothing to eat for two hours after the test meal so you can observe possible reactions.

The entire procedure is repeated on the next day.

Next, test other *fresh* meats such as pork and veal. The pork did not make Don hungry, but he felt tired and depressed after eating it, which meant that pork was incompatible with his chemistry. We crossed pork off his list of permissible meats.

Don had no difficulty after testing beef rib steaks, beef porterhouse steaks and veal chops. These gave him enough foods to form the central core of his diet. Accordingly, at each meal he ate beef rib steak, beef porterhouse steak or veal chops.

He ate half a cup of one fresh raw vegetable and one cup of fresh raw fruit after each meal as outlined earlier. We also started him on proper nutritional supplements.

Don lost 15 pounds the first week, then leveled off, losing two to three pounds a week. As warned, Don experienced more withdrawal symptoms. He got hungry for sweets. He turned restless, even more depressed and hostile.

"You don't know what you're doing. You're killing me!" he shouted.

Three more days and he was finished with all the withdrawal symptoms.

He reacted to celery. It gave him a headache. He reacted to lettuce. It sent him on another eating spree.

We posted 24-hour guards in case another test food (now fruits and vegetables) knocked out his appestat and made him want to spree eat.

Not only did he lost weight, but his blood pressure began falling. He had started off with a blood pressure of 190/110. It went down to 150/90. Within three more weeks it fell to 120/72. His arthritis and spastic colon completely cleared. This proved that they were, like his weight problem, only other manifestations of his food incompatibilities.

More importantly, he settled down and got his head back together again. He started rehearsals for his TV special and was delighted by how well they went.

Don was a people. People lack perfection.

Aside from his home, his clothes and his art, Don detested perfection. After his brilliant TV special, Don celebrated with champagne and went from there to ice cream, chocolate cake and cookies. In a single week he gained 42 pounds. (I'm sure part of this was fluid retention.) Soon the oily cloud of depression descended upon him. His colon trouble, his high blood pressure and his knee pain returned. This time he knew what to do. He went back on the diet.

Since then he has alternated between dieting and stuffing himself with carbohydrates. In all, he has lost about a hundred pounds. He could easily lose another hundred, but he is one of those persons who cannot long endure conformity. At least he learned what to do when he got into real trouble.

I've finally figured out why we can't be perfect.

You see, being God is a boring job. God made us imperfect so He could watch the never-ending soap operas that all of us live.

9

Different Ways on Different Days: The Dynamics of Food Incompatibilities

In the land of the blind, the one-eyed man is king.
—STREETS OF GOLD

Several years ago street-corner Santa Clauses were ringing Christmas bells. Warmly coated mothers and children stood in lines to look at the red, white and green moving figures in department store windows on Fifth Avenue. When I reached my office, I found a Christmas card from an allergist friend I hadn't heard from in years. I telephoned to thank him for the card and to chat about our mutual friends.

When I happened to mention food incompatibilities, he said, "You have to be careful about food reactions. They're tricky. Patients react to different foods in different ways on different days."

Although a well-qualified allergist, he, like most specialists in his field, does not understand food incompatibilities. Furthermore, he doesn't want to discuss the topic. He has a closed mind on the subject.

The sad thing is that he himself is suffering from a life-threatening food incompatibility. His blood pressure is seriously high. Sadly, the medication he takes to control his blood pressure leaves him tired, depressed and impotent. The chances are overwhelming that his high blood pressure is caused by an incompatibility with grains or table sugar.

Even though I've been able to cure every patient I've seen suffering

80

from high blood pressure by removing foods or other substances which were incompatible with their chemistries, he wouldn't listen to what I had to say about food incompatibilities.

My friend the allergist has died. People will readily die for a belief. Ask the crusaders and the men who followed Napoleon.

Most allergists view food incompatibilities as a mysterious land they don't understand. If they don't understand food incompatibilities, they think no one understands them.

Not true. The main reason that allergists don't understand food incompatibilities is that they fail to grasp the *dynamics* of food incompatibilities. They know a few things about *fixed* food incompatibilities, but they are not familiar with *cyclic* food incompatibilities.

Enzyme Systems

Our bodies combine a protein, one or more vitamins, and usually one or more minerals to make enzymes. Enzymes speed up the chemical reactions in the body. Without them, chemical reactions would be so slow we would die.

It's my theory that the body has a different enzyme system for handling each food. At least that's the way our body chemistry behaves. The body has one enzyme system for handling Red Delicious apples, another for Yellow Delicious apples, still a third for Granny Smith apples, and so on.

Because enzymes are made of vitamins, proteins and minerals, we are not stuck with the enzyme systems that we inherited. They can often be improved and made to work better (and thus leave us with fewer incompatibilities) if we consume ideal amounts of protein, vitamins and minerals.

Fixed Food Incompatibilities

If you have a *fixed food incompatibility*, you have an *absolute* deficiency in the enzyme system that handles a given food.

How do you discover whether you have a fixed incompatibility to a food?

If you eat only one food at a time, you'll find the answer. For a week do not eat the test food, say grapefruit. On the test day, for two hours before the test meal do not eat or drink anything (except water). Then eat a meal made of nothing but grapefruit. Eat nothing for two hours after the meal. Observe how you feel. Do you become hungry or do you experience a headache? Do you have gas or develop other symptoms? If you react unfavorably in any way to the food, you have a fixed food incompatibility to the test food. To double check for a fixed food incompatibility, wait for a month and repeat the test. If you react again, then clearly you have a *fixed* food incompatibility. You always react to grapefruit every time you eat it because you have a *fixed* food incompatibility with that food.

If you have a fixed food incompatibility, then you have an *absolute* deficiency in the enzyme system that's needed to metabolize that food. If your body lacks the enzyme systems needed to handle grapefruit, your body cannot use it. You may as well be eating axle grease.

During the time it takes your body to destroy and excrete the incompatible food, you will continue to react to it. Food reactions usually last three days, but sometimes go on for a week.

Don't forget that an incompatible food may strike any organ in the body. If it hits the *turn-off* cells in your appestat, it will send you on an eating spree.

Cyclic Food Incompatibilities

Cyclic food incompatibilities confuse allergists and weight losers alike.

If you do not react the first time you test a food, it may still be incompatible for you. You might have a cyclic rather than a fixed food incompatibility. To check whether you have a cyclic food incompatibility, test the food again the next day. Then test it again on the third day. An unfavorable reaction will not show up until the second or third time you test the food.

In working out food incompatibilities, people often eat (test) a food such as grapefruit. They have no reaction. They conclude that food is compatible for them. They mistakenly believe they can eat the food without harm. They begin eating the food every day or two. After a few days they become hungry—or have some other untoward reaction to the food—and don't understand why.

"It couldn't be the grapefruit," they think. "I tested the grapefruit and had no reaction to it."

Grapefruit is incompatible with their chemistry, however. *The reaction didn't show itself until they ate the food several times at close intervals.*

As noted, people with *fixed* incompatibilities have an *absolute deficiency* in the enzyme system they need to metabolize a certain food.

With *cyclic* food incompatibilities, however, the person has only a *relative deficiency* of the needed enzyme. The enzyme system is there, but it's weak. We must allow it to "rest" between the times we use it.

We can eat a food to which we have a cyclic food incompatibility without harm *if*:

We eat limited amounts of the food and space out the frequency with which we eat the food. That way our enzyme systems have time to recover between the times we use them.

I have a cyclic food incompatibility to grapefruit. If I eat one grapefruit every week, it makes me sleepy. If I eat one grapefruit every two weeks, it doesn't bother me.

Instead of feeling sleepy as a result of an incompatibility, you may become hungry.

I also have a cyclic food incompatibility to certain flavors and brands of ice cream. I can eat a small amount about once a month without reacting. I don't bother with it, however. It's less trouble for me—and probably will be for you—to let sleeping dogs sleep.

10

The World Is Out to Get You!

Life is a struggle between our biochemistry and the world in which we live.

—H. L. NEWBOLD

In spite of our awesome power and command over nature, today we are more threatened with death and destruction than ever before. Instead of crocodiles and lions, great industries listed on the stock exchange spend billions of dollars to sneak into our homes by way of small wires or electromagnetic waves that travel on airy nothingness. Psychologists have taught industries how to divert our attention so they can gobble away at our wallets—and our health.

How?

They play upon our primitive need for companionship, upon our love of colored pictures and the beat of music, and our fascination with other people and with bedtime stories. Then a cleverly worded "message from the sponsor" awakens within us a desire for foods and chemicals that are often incompatible with our chemistry.

Milk and breakfast cereals are equated with mother love. Beer is fellowship. Corn oil is a long and happy low-cholesterol life. A phenol-ammonia-chlorine sterilized home is a happy home.

Orwell's *1984* has arrived but not passed. The lie has become the truth. Repetition is the secret. Repeat a lie often enough and people will incorporate *the word* as the Gospel truth.

We are enticed to expose ourselves to foods and chemicals that make us ill with high blood pressure, arthritis, depression, fatigue, headaches and more than two dozen other common illnesses . . . and the foods addict us, knock out our appestats and make us overweight.

Chemicals

I'm sorry to tell you, but many things other than food can also disable our *turn-off* cells and, Dr. Jekyll and Mr. Hyde-like, change us into eating machines that won't stop.

We get hit by things like:

♦ Carpeting, which contains formaldehyde (plus dozens of other chemicals) some of which give people cancer as well as knock out many appestats and make people overweight.

♦ Copying machines and laser printers that blow into the air dozens of chemicals, including toxic levels of selenium. *Info World* has reported blindness from laser printers in Great Britain. Also, laser printers cause chest infections and other serious health problems. British Rail has delayed buying laser printers because of a lack of published safety standards. Even more serious, printers and copying machines send many people on eating sprees.

♦ Scented and perfumed cosmetics, hair and personal care items, soaps and cleansers.

♦ Household cleaning agents, gas from the kitchen stove—the list is endless. The items are a common part of "modern civilization."

This chapter and the next will help you identify and understand the unsuspected enemies that keep you from losing weight. *If you don't know that your hunger is caused by the chemicals in the diet soda you drink three times a day, trying to lose weight is like trying to learn to flap your hands and fly.*

You'll be happy to learn that not every spree eater has trouble with chemicals and other common substances. Among those who are troubled, often only one or two items are critical. Whether it be a food or gas from the kitchen stove, it's essential for us to spot the things that knock out the *turn-off* cells in our appestats.

Here's a *partial* list of some things in the environment (other than foods) that I've observed knocking out *turn-off* cells. My list keeps growing:

After-shave lotion

Alcoholic drinks in any form (very common)

Antihistamines

Antiperspirants

Aspirin (tablets contain corn, among other things)

Contraceptive jelly or foam

Chemicals (They surround us. Do you know that common paint has chemicals in it to kill mold?)

Cats, gerbils, and other pets (Very common, very serious, and very complicated. You can react from the cat's dander, from the oils that evaporate from the cat's skin. Also, you can react from the saliva, from the urine, the feces and the litter in the cat's box.)

Cockroaches

Coffee (Yes, even your old friend zero-calorie coffee can do you in and make you hungry.)

Coloring and flavoring agents in diet sodas

Condoms (The rubber, or the perfume in them, or the powder, or the lubricant some contain.)

Copy machines

Fire-retardant chemicals in mattresses

Flavoring in chewing gum

Foam mattresses

Foam rubber pillows

Food coloring

Fresh newsprint

Fumes from stop-and-go city traffic

Gas fumes from a kitchen stove (Now you know why you don't like to cook!)

House dust

Household cleaning products

Household deodorants

Insecticides

Laser printers
Laundry detergents
Laxatives
Lipstick
Mold (present in house plants, summer homes, cheeses)
Paper cups or paper milk cartons
Perfume
Plastics
Polyester pillows, comforters and clothes
Powder (cornstarch)
Perspiration (I've seen sensitive women who could not sleep with
    their husbands after they drank wine or smoked tobacco.)
Seminal fluid (I have had two women patients who reacted to some
    men's seminal fluid and not to others. It probably depended
    upon what the men ate, drank or smoked.)
Tobacco (Much more common than you suspect and complicated.
    Tobacco contains flavorings, molds, sprayed chemicals, insect
    parts, wood smoke and sugar from the curing process, chemi-
    cals in cigarette paper, hydrocarbons from lighter fluid.)
Toothpaste
Tranquilizers
Vaginal creams and douches
Vaginal secretions
Vitamins
Wallpaper and glues
Water (chlorides, fluorides, mold, etc.)

To make the connection between environmental triggers and overweight more understandable, let me tell you some of my reactions.

One afternoon I stopped by the apartment of a woman who typed
manuscripts. The moment I walked into the apartment, I smelled insect
spray. Because I'm very sensitive to insecticides, I made a quick retreat
and asked her to come out into the hall to talk. I explained that I was
sensitive to the spray she had used. We had a short discussion. Then
I left to walk to my apartment.

I had not gone half a block before I felt two things:

1. Depression.
2. A strong hunger for sweets.

Although depressed and hungry as a lion that has been living off celery for a week, I wasn't hungry for a steak and salad. Typical of hunger caused by incompatibilities, I wanted sweets. Nothing else would help.

I increased my pace and began walking as fast as possible. When tempted to pause and window-shop, I kept walking. After half an hour, the desire for sweets began fading. By the time an hour of hard walking passed, my compelling interest in sweets had vanished. My appestat had recovered from its assault.

Experience has taught me that depression and hunger for sweets are two of my toxic reactions.

Let me stress: incompatibilities may cause any symptom you can name—not just hunger. Although I develop depression and hunger from insecticides, I get tired from mushrooms. Some people develop tiredness, or arthritis, or high blood pressure.

People who are overweight, however, *commonly develop hunger as a reaction.* Often they get other reactions as well. Most overweight people know the enemy called *depression.* Usually depression is a symptom caused by exposure to a food or chemical that is incompatible with brain chemistry. People in this country, however, have been taught to blame their mates or fates. In other societies, people may blame the forest gods.

Cats, Gerbils and Other Pets

People think I dislike cats. Not true. In years past I've owned several cats. But not even the Census Bureau knows how many New Yorkers are sitting alone in their apartments on Saturday nights spree-eating ice cream because of an incompatibility with their cats.

A young lady with a weight problem visited my office. For a year I've been telling her that I suspect her mother's cats are defeating her attempt to take off pounds and inches. Recently she left home and got her own apartment. Her appetite has lessened and at last she's begun to win her battle.

"I think you're right about the cats," she admitted. "Every time I go home I go on an eating spree."

My biggest problem is that patients don't believe what I tell them. No one is more critical of my findings than I. I know what I know because

I've learned from my reactions and the reactions of all the patients who have visited my office.

Sometimes I tell a patient, "Look, let's play a game. Let's pretend I know more about this than you do. Do as I say, and let's see what happens."

Tobacco

The late Roger Williams, professor of chemistry at the University of Texas, stated that smoking tobacco often injures either the *turn-off* cells or the *turn-on* cells. I have had patients made hungry either when they smoke or when they expose themselves to smoke from other people's tobacco.

On the other hand, many people who smoke lose their appetites and stay underweight. You know friends who gained weight after they stopped smoking. That's because they substituted one addiction for another. They give up tobacco, but develop an addiction to sweets.

This substitution of addictions is common. I've spoken at AA groups. Nowhere is substitute addiction more evident. Cookies, coffee and cigarettes abound.

The withdrawal symptoms people feel when they stop smoking—or drop other addictions—make them crave sweets. The good news is, *if they resist the craving for sweets for four days, the craving will lessen and soon vanish.*

Marijuana frequently brings on a compelling desire to eat sweets. The hunger comes from an incompatibility with the marijuana plant, a grain.

You've already learned that your favorite food is the one to which you're incompatible. Ironically, the same is often true of your favorite indulgence.

If your chemistry is incompatible with marijuana, you will probably like it. If you're incompatible to grapes, you'll probably fall in love with wine. It will give you that special send-off you can find nowhere else. On the other hand, if you're incompatible with corn and rye, bourbon will probably be your thing.

The Christmas Environment

Christmas assaults many people with incompatibilities.

I felt especially lonely during Christmas many years ago when I first moved to New York. I knew no one in New York. Seeking fellowship, I went to church. The fresh scent of a pine forest greeted me. Boughs of evergreens decorated the altar, along with colorful flowers. Women wore not only their new Christmas dresses, but also their new Christmas perfumes.

The scent from the evergreens, the flowers and the perfumes was too much. I developed an uncontrollable hunger and had to leave. I felt like raiding pastry shops and gobbling down all the Christmas goodies in Manhattan.

Christmas-New Year's parties may assault me—and you!—savagely.

Usually I can handle parties if too many people aren't jammed into too small a space. The best parties for me are penthouse parties on the patio or lawn parties where a breeze moves in off the Long Island Sound.

These items in the environment attacked me last New Year's Eve when I went to a party:

1. A ceiling-high spruce Christmas tree.
2. Perfume (men and women)
3. Large candles that filled the apartment with hydrocarbons, carbon dioxide and a mixture of burning wax and incense.
4. "Air freshener," a chemical spray to make the apartment "smell fresh."
5. Wall-to-wall carpet "cleaned" (chemicalized) for the holidays. Also, the carpet was coated with chemicals to mothproof it. They then coated it with chemicals to protect it from "soil." (Few people realize that chemicals themselves are, next to radioactive contamination, the worst possible "soil.")
6. Of course the guests soon filled the apartment with cigarette smoke, allowing me to play a game called "Russian Roulette Cancer."

To protect myself, I eased over to the terrace door and stepped outside for a few deep breaths. Even the New York City air tasted fresh and pure in comparison.

Finally, I left the party and went for a fast walk. That night, every sidewalk in Manhattan led to an ice cream shop. Fortunately, their lights were off and their doors were locked.

Parenthetically, have you ever noticed how extra crazy everybody gets during the Christmas season? You and your friends feel gloomy and depressed. Mates fight. Cab drivers and salespeople jump down your throat. It's a well recognized syndrome called "Christmas neurosis."

Every Christmas season I see psychologists on TV speaking about holiday depression. Not trained in the biological sciences and in biochemistry, psychologists make up fairy tales to explain the Christmas neurosis. No, they don't blame the forest gods. They talk about the Viennese gods and blame our "psychology," our mates and our fates. They say that people's longing for childhood and the time when we received without having to give is stirred up by the Christmas season.

Not true. Like almost all emotional difficulties, the Christmas neurosis purely and simply results from biochemical insults that impinge upon the brain's biochemistry. People overeat on incompatible foods and overdrink on incompatible drinks and are exposed to added environmental insults such as resin from Christmas trees. (On Earth Day we plant trees. To celebrate Christ's birthday, we cut them down!)

Dust

Always suspect dust intolerance when you are unable to control your eating. It's especially common during winter months.

Drs. Herbert Rinkel, Theron Randolph and Michael Zeller mentioned in their book *Food Allergy* that 90 percent of the people with food incompatibilities also have dust intolerance. I suspect the figure is 100 percent.

Office Dangers

As we continue adding more chemicals to the workplace, good ventilation becomes ever more important. As mentioned earlier, commonplace things like polyester carpeting, copying machines, and laser printers give off chemicals that will knock out your *turn-off* cells and send people on an eating spree.

Wallpaper is a frequent threat at work, as are plants and the filters used in air conditioners. The ink in fresh print strikes some people.

Not long ago I had a patient who could hardly squeeze into the generous visitor's chair in my inner office. Her weight had not been a problem until she finished designers' school and started working in Manhattan's garment industry. She sat in a small, dusty office piled high with reams of cloth. She could not tolerate the polyester, the formaldehyde or some dyes. Models wearing perfume walked in and out of the rooms, and cigar- and cigarette-smoking buyers inspected the goods.

A psychiatrist would say that the pressures of functioning as an adult were too much for her and would further pontificate that to offset her anxiety, the patient began eating excessively and became overweight.

Not true. Controlled exposure proved that her eating resulted from an intolerance to her environment. Dust, we found, not only made her hungry but gave her palpitations and almost made her faint.

We tried to ventilate her office so she could keep working at her profession. She remained a designer, but had to change to a different environment in the industry.

Other Threats

Odors from cooking foods, as mentioned earlier, often send people on eating sprees or make them react in other ways. If you cook, be especially watchful. Suspect gas from the kitchen stove. The gas gets not only into the air but into the food cooked in the oven. For example, a steak broiled under gas gives me an immediate reaction. Remember, gas is a hydrocarbon and hydrocarbons are carcinogenic. I don't want hydrocarbons in my home, thank you.

Cockroaches, mice and other pests are also a threat.

Diet Drinks

Again, be warned about your close friend, diet soda. Sodas contain food coloring and other chemicals. They send many people on eating sprees and make them gain extra pounds.

I was delighted to learn about an article published by the American

Cancer Society. They studied 80,000 women, most of whom *gained* weight when drinking diet sodas.

Any chemical used in processing foods could send you on an eating spree. Weight loss may be impossible for the person who eats such foods.

Here's a partial list of chemicals commonly added to processed foods:

Anticaking agents, free-flow agents
Antimicrobial agents
Antioxidants
Colors, coloring adjuncts (color stabilizers, color fixatives, color retentive agents, etc.)
Curing, pickling agents
Dough strengtheners
Drying agents
Emulsifiers, emulsifier salts
Enzymes
Firming agents
Flavor enhancers
Flavoring agents, adjutants
Flour-treating agents (including bleaching and maturing agents)
Formulation aids (carriers, binders, fillers, plasticizers, film-formers, tableting aids)
Fumigants
Humectants, moisture-retention agents, antidusting agents
Leavening agents
Lubricants, release agents
Nonnutritive sweeteners
Nutrient supplements
Nutritive sweeteners
Oxidizing and reducing agents
pH control agents (including buffers, acids, alkalies, neutralizing agents)
Processing aids (including clarifying agents, clouding agents, catalysts, flocculents, filter aids, etc.)
Propellants,aerating agents, gases sequestrants
Solvents, vehicles

Stabilizers, thickeners (suspending and bodying agents, setting agents, gelling agents, bulking agents)

Surface-active agents (other than emulsifiers, including solubilizing agents, dispersants, detergents, wetting agents, rehydration enhancers, whipping agents, foaming agents, defoaming agents)

Surface-finishing agents (including glazes, polishes, waxes, protective coatings)

Synergists (chemicals which make two incompatible substances work together. For example, a synergist might be needed if a chef uses olive oil and water together.)

Texturizers

When Is an Apple Not an Apple?

These chemicals are allowed in *apple flavoring*. You can imagine how long the list would be if we included all flavorings used by food processors!

Chemical compounds used to make *apple flavoring*:

Acetaldehyde
Acetic acid
Acetone
Acetophenone
Benzoic acid
Benzyl acetate
Butanal
Butanol
2-Butanone
1-Butoxy-1-ethoxyethane
Butyl acetate
Butyl butyrate
Butyl hexanoate
Butyl propionate
Butyric acid
Diacetyl
1,1-Diethoxyethane
Formaldehyde
Formic acid
Furfural

Diethyl ether
Ethanol
1-Ethoxy-1-hexoxyethane
1-Ethoxy-1-methoxyethane
1-Ethoxy-1-(2-methylbutoxy) ethane
1-Ethoxy-1-propoxyethane
Ethyl acetate
Ethyl butyrate
Ethyl formate
Ethyinexanoate
Ethyl-2-methylbutyrate
Ethyl-2-methylpropionate
Ethyl octanoate
Ethyl pentanoate
Ethyl-2-phenylacetate
Ethyl propionate
2-Methyl propane
Methyl-propane-1-ol
2-Methyl propionic acid

Geraniol

Hexanal

Hexanoic acid

n-Hexanoic acid

2-Hexanone

2-Hexenal, trans

2-Hexen-1-ol, trans

2-Hexenyl acetate, trans

Isobutanol

Isopentane

Methanol

2-Methylbutanal

3-Methylbutanal

2-Methylbutane-1-ol

3-Methylbutane-1-ol

Methyl butyrate

3-Methylbutyric acid

Methyl formate

Methyl hexanoate

Methyl 2-methylbutyrate

Methyl 3-methylbutyrate

1-Methyl-naphthalene

2-Methyl-naphthalene

2-Methylpropyl acetate

2-Methylpropyl propionate

Nonanal

Pentanal

Pentanoic acid

2-Pentanone

3-Pentanone

Pentyiacetate

Pentyl butyrate

Pentyl-2-methylbutyrate

2-Phenylethyl acetate

Propanal

Propanol

2-Propanol

Propionaldehyde

Propionic acid

Propyl acetate

2-Propyl acetate

Propyl butyrate

Propyl pentanoate

Propyl propionate

2,4,5-trimethyl-1,

3-dioxoiane

We're lost if we put ourselves at the mercy of the food manufacturers.

Now do you understand why I ask overweight patients to start by eating only primary foods? Primary foods are simple, unprocessed foods. Examples: *fresh* fish-fowl-meat-vegetable-fruit.

Years From Now

"Primitive and naive." Two hundred years from now that's how they'll describe those of us who lived back in the 20th century.

Why?

We've discovered tens of thousands of chemicals that work wonders, but we've done little to learn how to live with the chemicals without having them attack us. Even the conservative American Cancer Society admits that 70 percent of cancer is manmade.

Why doesn't anyone do anything to prevent cancer? There's no money in preventing cancer. On the other hand, multimillion-dollar grants are handed out to those who treat cancer.

I look out of my office window and see a deadly chemical filth in the form of smoke billowing from the smokestacks of New York, including some buildings owned by the city of New York. Pouring smoke into the air is illegal, but no one enforces the law. Why? If a D.A. "fights crime" he gets his name in the papers as a good guy. With luck the publicity might move him into the governor's chair. If he plays it right, he might go from governor to president.

Whoever got elected by fighting air pollution?

When I realize that recently we spent $15 million a month keeping oil-carrying ships safe in the Persian gulf, I cannot help wondering why we fight for oil when it will only give us cancer—and obesity! Why aren't we spending that money to develop solar energy?

Politicians can get elected by fighting Iraq.

Politicians can't get elected to the school board in Pascagoula on a platform advocating solar energy.

So what do I do, live in a cave and eat deer? Not at all. Soon you'll know the secrets for living easily and conveniently in the world of today while sidestepping threats that may cause weight problems and other serious conditions.

11

How to Test For and Avoid Environmental Threats

> *Small is the number of them that see with their own eyes and feel with their own hearts.*
> —EINSTEIN

First Step: Be Suspicious

Most people are great detectives once they become suspicious. They easily discover the threats lurking all around them.

Anyone who has had trouble following a weight-loss program in the past should pay close attention to environmental threats. Most people cheat because they have the *turn-off* cells in their appestat knocked out by an incompatibility. When your *turn-off* cells are damaged, you may not have dramatic eating sprees. Instead you may have multiple mini eating sprees throughout the day.

After I appear on a radio or TV talk show, people often write to me. They never imagined that gas from the kitchen stove or tobacco or insecticides could make them feel as hungry as a bear coming out of hibernation. Suddenly, people begin discovering incompatibilities that they never dreamed existed.

It's the same with patients in my office. After spotting a few reactions, they quickly add to their list.

Second Step: Keep a Diary

Write down each of your activities and record how you feel during each part of the day for at least one week. You'll do a better job of record-keeping if you buy a bound notebook. Write the day of the week and the date at the top of each page. Use a new page for each day. Next, divide the day into two-hour sections. Write the time on the left-hand margin of the page.

Always carry the notebook with you. Every two hours, jot down a sentence or two about what you've been doing and what you've been eating. Comment on your hunger and note how you feel. Here's a brief sample of how your record might look:

Tuesday, June 2

7:00 a.m.	Got up feeling great. Toast, marmalade and coffee for breakfast.
9:00 a.m.	Tired and hungry after breakfast. Ate a doughnut and took a nap.
11:00 a.m.	Better, especially after a walk to the grocery store.
1:00 p.m.	Headache on the elevator. Felt grouchy. Suddenly hungry.
3:00 p.m.	Was feeling better until I visited a department store. Got very hungry. Took a walk to fight off the temptation to eat.
5:00 p.m.	Recovered. Visited Ruth and her new kittens. Uncontrollably hungry. Ate two cheese blintzes. Still starving. Had a pecan pie à la mode. Headache and felt blah.
7:00 p.m.	Hungry and tired after cooking and serving dinner. Didn't eat. I'm depressed and discouraged. Nothing will ever help me lost weight!
9:00 p.m.	Dozed off while watching favorite TV program. Now I'm beginning to wake up.
11:00 p.m.	Feel better than I've felt at any time since I got up. Wish it weren't bedtime.

Third Step: Analyze the Information

If you got up feeling like a million, that probably means that your body chemistry is compatible with your mattress, pillow, sheets and blankets.

You turned tired and hungry after breakfast. Both tiredness and hunger are symptoms of incompatibility. Whenever symptoms follow a meal, note what you ate before your symptoms started. You had toast, marmalade and coffee.

All three of these foods are often trouble makers and could give you symptoms. On the other hand, you cooked eggs and oatmeal for the rest of your family. Could gas from the kitchen stove have caused your reaction?

On the following morning, cook breakfast for your family and have nothing to eat yourself. It will help you learn whether you're reacting to breakfast or to the gas.

Note that you got a headache, felt grouchy, and became hungry while on the elevator. What happened on the elevator? Nothing that you can remember. Was anyone else on the elevator with you? Oh, yes, Mrs. Cardington. She always wears so much perfume you can smell her a block away and she lives with a cigarette between her fingers.

Perfume and *cigarettes* are the key words. Did either of them cause a reaction and make you hungry? Remember to test them separately and learn the answer.

The next time you felt bad, you were in a department store. What did you buy? Eye shadow. In which department? Cosmetics, of course. What could have set you off there? Ah, perfume again. The place smelled like a harem.

You became uncontrollably hungry after visiting Ruth. Ruth doesn't smoke. She never wears perfume during the day. What could have caused trouble? Cats were on the list. You didn't feel hungry until you lifted one of the kittens and held it to your face!

It's not fair, reacting to something as innocent as a kitten!

Symptoms came on again after supper. Gas from the kitchen stove again?

Back in the 1960s when I first saw Theron Randolph's film on incompatibilities to items common to our everyday lives, my reaction was, "This is too complicated. Just stand me against the wall and shoot me."

At first it seems like a tough battle, but if you'll use your intelligence and persist, you'll win. Don't expect to solve all the problems at once. Look upon discovering your chemical relationship to the world as a hobby. It's your personal detective story. The only difference is, you're looking for *what* did it rather than *who* did it.

Test Yourself

Always consult with and follow the advice of your physician before testing yourself. Be especially cautious if you suffer from such classical allergies as hay fever, hives or asthma. Be careful not to give yourself too large a test dose.

Wait until you're feeling good. Have a sniff of perfume or ask a friend to blow some cigarette smoke your way. That's provocative testing at its best. It's inexpensive. It's better testing than you can buy at any laboratory or doctor's office. The only problem with this type of testing: It doesn't help the doctor pay his rent.

Expose yourself to other suspected offenders. If you wonder about dust, shake a dust mop near your face. Bleach you use in your laundry? Place a few drops on a paper towel and fan some of the fumes in your direction.

Life Is a Test

You may walk into a friend's house and find her airing winter clothes. The odor from the mothballs might knock out your *turn-off* cells and make you want to speed to the shopping mall for a double ice cream sundae. You might get a whiff of phenol in the detergent used to scrub an office floor. The chef at a restaurant might decide to flavor your steak with a dash of MSG.

The more you learn about incompatibilities, the fewer surprises you'll get.

As noted earlier, tobacco gives many exposures. It includes cyanide, dead mold, sugar and wood smoke (from the curing process), and parts of insects and chemical sprays.

By far the best way to break an addiction to tobacco is to go on a water fast for four days. During that time, the only thing you take by mouth is water and air. You absolutely must not have one puff of tobacco; otherwise, this very effective method won't work.

Overweight people should not own pets; especially they should not own gerbils, rabbits, birds and *cats*. Pets often cause classical reactions such as a stuffy nose or asthma. Commonly they also disrupt the brain's chemistry and make people fatigued, depressed, tense, forgetful, poor achievers in school and in life—and make them overweight.

Dogs give fewer reactions than cats. I've found poodles and Akitas give the least trouble. In my experience the length of the hair has nothing to do with whether a pet causes a reaction.

Desensitization shots are not satisfactory. The dander is not the most common problem. The skin oils that vaporize and enter the air cause more trouble. Also, people may react to one cat or dog but not to another. Skin testing for animal's dander wastes time and money. Not only might you react to one cat and not to another, but your appestat might react when your skin fails to react.

It's much better to make other permanent living arrangements for your cat or dog. This is true especially of cats. Even if you have the pet live somewhere else for three to six months, it will be helpful. In that period you will be able to clear most traces of the animal from your clothes and home. Then you can have several controlled exposures to the animal and better learn whether it is one of your problems. Do not, however, send it to live where there are other animals. That will interfere with your testing.

No matter what you do to lose weight, an incompatibility with your pet may well defeat you and condemn you to remaining overweight. At the moment, I can't remember a single patient with a cat who lost weight and kept it off—unless they gave up their cat or reduced their exposure to the cat by following the directions given below.

When the owner cannot give up a cat or dog, here are ways to reduce exposure. But you must realize that reducing exposure is second-best and considerable trouble. Here's how:

1. The bedroom door must always remain closed and the owner must never allow the pet in the bedroom. Keep the bedroom window cracked open.
2. Shower and shampoo each night before going to bed. Have no contact with your pet or with the contaminated part of your home after bathing.

3. The owner must wash the pet with warm water and a non-scented shampoo once a week. Soak the animal with warm water. Work up heavy suds. Rinse with warm water. Repeat the wash.

   Sometimes cats are reluctant to allow bathing. It may be necessary to tape their front paws together. Then tape their rear paws. Use adhesive tape. Some patients find it easier to bathe their cats if they stand a window screen securely in the tub and allow the cat to cling to the wire.

4. After washing your pet, apply Dust Seal* to your pet to hold down the shedding of dander. Repeat once a week. Dust Seal is the brand name of the product. Follow the directions on the label and mix Dust Seal with water before applying. Apply with a sponge. *Do not spray.* If you spray it, you might inhale droplets. Lungs and inhaled fat droplets do not get on well together.

   Before using Dust Seal, you must test it to make certain that it's not incompatible with your biochemistry. I've seen only one patient who reacted to Dust Seal; still, it's best to be careful. To test Dust Seal, dilute some of it according to directions. Use a sponge to apply it to a reasonably clean, old, all-cotton towel. Hang the towel up to dry in the air. After the towel is dry, drape it across your pillow and sleep on it for a couple of nights. If the Dust Seal is incompatible with your body chemistry, the incompatibility gods will communicate with you.

5. After washing and Dust Sealing your pet for the first time, clean your home thoroughly. Go over everything with damp paper towels to remove all dust and dander. Give special attention to the floors, walls, ceilings, above door frames, picture frames, etc.

   Air your home well and keep it aired out.

   Dust Seal all the fabric in your home to reduce the dander in the air. Apply it to *all* fabrics: mattresses (front, sides, and back, including the box springs), mattress covers, blankets. Because you wash them often, you may omit the sheets. Apply the Dust Seal to draperies, rugs, and carpets, upholstered furniture, pillows, stuffed toys—everything covered with fabric.

   You'll be happy to learn that you need to reapply Dust

---

*Available from Wilner Chemists, 330 Lexington Avenue, New York, NY 10016; 212 685-0448.

Seal to fabrics only every five years. If you wash them, however, reapply Dust Seal.

   To rid them of dander and vaporized oils from your pet, wash or clean all of your clothes. Also, wash or clean all of the clothes belonging to everyone else in your household. Include the clothes of your intimate friends. For example, if you have been spending one night a week with your boyfriend, you have seeded his clothes and apartment with cat contamination.

6. You can usually make dogs and cats *much* less incompatible if you change their diets. Different foods give a different composition to their saliva, urine, feces, and—especially—skin oils. I've had no firsthand experience so I cannot say whether you can make other pets such as gerbils and parrots less allergenic by changing their diets.

   You should switch the diet of dogs and cats *gradually* to a mostly meat diet. Beef is usually best. *The meat must contain fat, otherwise your pet will starve.* Small chunks of raw meat are best.

   Some dogs and cats will enjoy a vegetable now and then. Try a leaf of lettuce or a bit of carrot.

   Feed raw liver (but not raw pork liver) twice a week for vitamins. Do not give your pet B vitamins. Most contain yeast, even those labeled "yeast free." Add half a kelp tablet once or twice a week for trace minerals. Mix some dolomite powder and zinc gluconate powder with the meat. Add cod liver oil, safflower and linseed (flaxseed) oil. (Buy the linseed oil at a health food store, *not* at a hardware or paint store!)

The amount of supplements will vary with the age and weight of your pet.

Seek your veterinarian's advice. Remember, however, that your veterinarian is not likely to know about incompatibilities. Especially is he or she unlikely to be familiar with the newer aspects of incompatibilities such those discussed in this book.

He might mistakenly try to discourage you from carrying out your project. Both physicians and veterinarians who are unfamiliar with something tend to puff up, pontificate and condemn it.

Friends who own pets can be a problem. In the early part of your program, don't visit friends who have pets and don't allow them in your home. It's better—especially if the friend has a gerbil, cat, bird or rabbit—to meet in the park. Sit on one end of the bench and have your friend sit, down wind, on the other end. Pretend they're radioactive!

With a little luck you will lose pet-owning friends. Sorry, it just doesn't work out.

Sometimes we don't like the choices life forces upon us. I don't like paying taxes so politicians can drive around in chauffeured limousines. On the other hand, I don't think I would like prison life.

Bare Is Beautiful!

If you find that your biochemistry is incompatible with many common chemicals, keep everything possible out of your office and home. This includes pets and people who own pets, perfume, gas, kerosene and woodburning stoves.

You will probably do better without carpeting, flowers and plants. You should be especially suspicious of scented and unscented beauty products, and of people who smoke.

Your bedroom should be your special haven. Strip it of everything except a metal bed frame and your mattress. You should cover your mattress with several layers of all-cotton barrier cloth or flannel.

Furniture is a problem, often because it has backing made of particle board that outgases formaldehyde. Plywood also has formaldehyde in it.

If you're extremely incompatible with many chemicals, keep the temperature down in your home, keep the air humid and reduce the dust as much as possible. Books (dust, mold, print, paper) belong in closed bookcases.

Incidentally, if you humidify your home, don't use city water. When it evaporates, it puts chlorine into the air, which might make you hungry and give you weight problems. Use a *steam* humidifier.

The humidifiers that jet out a cool mist have mold growing in places that are inaccessible for cleaning. They spray mold into the air that might well send you on an eating spree. Also, they might give you a mold pneumonia.

If anyone asks why you're throwing away your carpeting, tell them it's part of your new weight-reducing program. I promise an interesting discussion.

Dust from fabrics can cause trouble. The dust contains mites, a tiny insect. They're in carpets, draperies, stuffed furniture, automobile seats, mattresses, box springs, pillows, mattress pads—in any fabric that's not often washed. The mite leaves the fabric, gets into the air in the form of dust and spreads about the house, the cells in your nose, or in your lungs. Also, a reaction to them might knock out your appestat.

Heating Problems

In the wintertime dust lands on the radiators or electrical heating elements. The heat fries the dust and sends it back into the air as smaller particles that cause trouble. Forced-air heat blows dust about. A filter helps. Avoid electrostatic and fiberglass filters. The electrostatic filters often put ozone in the air. Even minute traces of ozone are toxic. Fiberglass filters are oil-treated to make them catch dust more efficiently. Many people develop an allergic reaction to the traces of the oil.

A heat pump outside of the house is often a good solution for both heating and cooling.

A gas- or oil-burning furnace (or hot-water heater) may cause trouble for many people. You can mount a fan in the flue that will usually solve the problem.

Even if living in a 150-room castle, people spend most of their time in one or two rooms. It's a good idea to turn the heat down. The room you occupy can ideally be heated with several 250-watt infrared bulbs such as those made by G.E. Dust the bulbs frequently.

Full-Spectrum Light

"The wrong light makes me overweight? Come on, you've got to be kidding!"

I kid you not. I've had patients who were incompatible with a food only when they eat the food under artificial light. Ordinary fluorescent light is the biggest troublemaker.

Most people need full-spectrum light. That's the type of light you get outdoors. Also, you want full-spectrum lenses for your glasses. Soft contact lenses are full-spectrum. Only a few places sell full-spectrum hard contact lenses.

Many stores sell full-spectrum fluorescent tubes. Their trade name is Vita Lite. If you have trouble finding them, try Rosetta Electric, 21 West 46th Street, New York, New York 10036 1-212-719-4381.

Now do you know why you never lost weight and kept it off?

Note: Don't let someone talk you into a "full-spectrum" bulb. I haven't run scientific tests on them, but I've tried them. Something's wrong with them.

Good News

Remember, most overweight people react to only a few items. Again, your biggest problems are likely to be: cats, gas from the kitchen stove, household cleaning products, indoor plants, non-cotton pillows, perfumed products, tobacco and wall-to-wall carpeting.

Don't be discouraged. Armed with knowledge for the first time, you now have a fighting chance.

12

Special Ways to Fight *Type-A* and *Type-B* Weight Problems

All of us—poor man, rich man, beggar man, thief— are dancing to a tune played by evolution.

—H. L. NEWBOLD

How to Prevent Eating Sprees (Type-A)

First: Make certain that you have no nutritional deficiencies. Take proper vitamins, minerals, and unsaturated oils.

Second: Make sure you're eating enough animal fat and that you are not mistaking plain hunger for spree eating.

Third: Discover what knocks out the *Turn-Off* cells in your appestat.

Chapter Eight tells how to test yourself for foods that usually knock out the *Turn-Off* cells in your appestat.

Chapter 11 tells how to test for things in your home or office that trigger spree eating.

How to Block an Eating Spree

When a desire to spree eat strikes, it's a medical emergency. Eating sprees are a threat to you. To save your life, you must learn how to stop the desire to spree eat.

If you're an unusually tough character, you may be able to simply ride out your strong desire to eat. You might be able to hang on to the bedpost and wait for the urge to pass. Most of us can't do that. Here are some easier ways to block your drive to eat.

Walk!

A fast one-hour walk is one of the surest and cheapest ways to kill the urge to spree eat. There's something about the act of walking that settles the body chemistry. Our ancestors have been walking upright for four million years. Our body chemistry has come to depend upon the jarring motion of walking. (More about that in Chapter 22.) Not only will a good hard hour's walk often stop the desire to spree eat, but people who walk regularly become less reactive.

If you can't walk, crawl!

A Formula

Take nothing without your physician's approval! The following formula helps most people block an eating spree:
1. Place one teaspoon of ascorbic acid powder (fine) in a full glass of room-temperature water.
2. Add two tablets of Alka-Seltzer *Gold. This is not the regular Alka-Seltzer in the blue package.* Allow the tablets to dissolve. These Alka-Seltzer tablets contain nothing other than an effervescent antacid formula.
3. When you drink the mixture, also take two 250-mg L-carnitine capsules; two 218-mg calcium pantothenate capsules; three 200-mg vitamin B6 capsules; two 60-mg zinc gluconate capsules; and two 250-mg magnesium oxide tablets.
4. At the same time take two Bufferin tablets.

Many popular over-the-counter medications help lessen reactions from incompatibilities. Incompatibilities are behind most common disorders such as upset stomach, backache, muscular aches, headaches, arthritis, depression, the blahs, and many more. People have learned that they get relief from these popular products.

5. Walk around the block a few times until the remedies you take start working. Better still, walk for a full hour.

No matter how you stop an eating spree (even if you simply sweat it out), it's always a good idea to go someplace else.

For example, if you are sitting home and a strong need to spree eat strikes you, get out of the house. Go for a walk. See a movie. Visit the library. Buy a new dress or shirt. Start doing something different.

If Ready to Kill

If you feel like you absolutely will jump out of your cotton-pickin' mind if you don't spree eat, cheat by eating fresh fruits. Never, *ever* cheat with anything that contains alcohol, chocolate, grains, table sugar, honey, milk or nuts. Mind you, I didn't tell you to cheat. I said, if you're going to either cheat or turn into a Rambo and mow down half the town, cheat by eating *fresh* fruit.

If the desire to spree eat keeps returning, you're missing something. You're drinking water which is not compatible with your chemistry or eating an incompatible food. You may be reacting to cooking odors. Perhaps you're reacting to something you haven't identified in your home or office. You may be addicted to a food and be having repeated withdrawal reactions. Possibly your appestat is not working properly because you aren't on the right vitamins, minerals and unsaturated fats. Possibly one of your nutritional supplements is not compatible with your chemistry. Read the chapters that cover those problems. Observe, think and solve your problems.

Addictive Eating (Type-B)

Addiction to foods causes much more harm than addictions to narcotics such as cocaine and heroin.

Food addictions cause people to be overweight. They also cause illnesses like insomnia, depression, tiredness, high blood pressure, arthritis, migraine, duodenal ulcers, lupus, scleroderma and many others.

Two hundred years from now people will smile sadly when they speak of their ignorant 20th century ancestors. They'll wonder why we jailed people caught selling cocaine and heroin, but allowed people selling sugar, wheat, milk products, nuts and chocolate to go free.

If you *must* cheat by eating a certain food, you are addicted to it. You will never lose weight and keep it off until you get off that particular food. Getting off the food is difficult. You have withdrawal symptoms when you leave off the food. The withdrawal can be as painful as the withdrawal from narcotics.

The same things that help block eating sprees also ease withdrawal illness.

Refer above to the information about blocking eating sprees.

In addition, you might have your physician give you a few Valium tablets. Never take Valium for more than two days. It's *very* addictive. Leaving off wheat and taking up Valium is not progress!

Injections of vitamin B12 often help. You might need an injection of vitamin B12 several times a day for a few days. *Careful: If you get too much B12, you might become hyperactive and be unable to sleep.* Some people are allergic to B12. Your physician should give you several small (0.1 cc to 0.3 cc) doses of the 1000 mcg/dl strength to make certain you aren't allergic to it. You may need three to nine cc to stop your withdrawal illness.

Although nothing is beneficial for everyone, people rarely feel worse on B12. The hydroxocobalamin (vitamin B12b) is the preferred form, as opposed to cyanocobalamin. If your physician has trouble finding hydroxocobalamin, he may order it from: Henry Schein, Inc., Port Washington, NY, or from Lypomed, Inc., Melrose Park, IL.

Last Resort

If you cannot leave off the foods that have addicted you, ask your physician for permission to go on a four-day fast. If he approves, go on a four-day water fast. Eat nothing. Drink only water for four days. At the end of the fourth day, you will be free of your addictive food. (Fasting is the only way many people can stop using tobacco.)

Some people can go about their day and do light work while fasting. Many people have marked withdrawal symptoms. Do not perform dangerous acts while fasting. For example, don't drive a car or a tractor. Don't use an engine-driven saw or lawn mower. Have a person with you if you feel the least bit faint.

Alcoholism is only a form of food addiction. Ask an AA member what happens when a "recovered" alcoholic starts drinking again. The member will tell you that the former alcoholic will again become an alcoholic.

It's best not to return to the food that addicted to you. You might be able to, but it's dangerous. See Chapter 25 on cheating. What if you become addicted again? Go on another fast and start all over again.

Persistence is the only horse that wins!

Remember, the second day of withdrawal is usually the worst.

If you continue craving the addictive food, something in your home or office is knocking out your appestat. That can explain why you crave carbohydrates. Your chemistry might be incompatible with your mink coat or your boyfriend's after-shave or the wrong type of light at work.

13

Cooking's No Hassle

Marriage is a step in the dark.
> —MRS. PEACOCK, CIRCA 1920

Eating in a restaurant is a step in the dark.
> —DR. NEWBOLD, CIRCA 1980

I would have laughed in his face if anyone in medical school had told me that one day I would write a chapter on how to cook. I don't like to cook—I never did. If cooking were not so important for me and other people with multiple food incompatibilities, I would never have learned. As the fates would have it, however, I've become an expert cook. I'm so good I can teach you to cook all of your food and spend less than 20 minutes a week at it. (Make that 23 minutes if you include cleaning up.)

The Fun-Food Trap

This book would bring in more money if I promised that you could eat chocolate mousse for breakfast, ice cream for lunch and apple pie for dinner—and lose weight.

I would, however, be earning dirty money. Dirty money brings nothing but trouble. I want to write an honest book that scientists will read 200 years from now, nod their heads and say, "You know, Newbold was right. He understood weight problems better than anyone else."

It's relatively easy to become rich. You only need to tell people what they want to hear. Picking up a slice of immortality is more difficult—and more valuable.

Once you start eating for pleasure, you're lost.

It's not a sensuous pleasure when you fill your car's gas tank. You fill the tank so you can use the car for work, or to drive yourself to the beach and enjoy yourself. Overweight people need to learn to take in food simply to make their human machine go.

Making food taste better is a mistake. Those of us with weight problems must not eat for pleasure. We must eat to feel buoyantly good and to be able to work hard and still have the energy left for away-from-the-table pleasures.

When we stop having pleasure at the table, we feel a pleasure vacuum. To fill the vacuum, we need to start new activities. I write books. You may need to start a mail-order business or begin growing your own vegetables. Somehow you need to find a way to get your pleasures away from the table.

Danger!

If you have a mental picture of overflowing baskets of health-giving green, yellow and red fruits and vegetables, put it aside. Unless you grow your own fruits and vegetables and know their history, they are as full of chemicals as a chemist's dictionary. In truth, no one knows what long-term effects the chemicals will have on you—or on your children or your children's children.

When companies develop a new dog food, they test it for at least three generations before putting it on the market. Why? Because that's how long it takes for some dietary defects to show themselves.

"But the FDA protects me from harmful chemicals!" you protest.

Did it protect you from DDT and PCBs? Did it protect you from tampons and toxic shock syndrome? Look, the government is primarily interested in protecting itself. If it tried to pass logical laws against fruit and vegetable farmers, tobacco farmers, and milk producers, the government would be besieged by special interest groups. Senators and congressmen would be threatened with the loss of their next election. Many of them couldn't earn a living any other way.

The government's interest in protecting you is secondary.

Besides, even if fruits and vegetables were perfect, many people trying to lose weight would not thrive on them. Vegetables and fruits must be eaten only in small amounts. They are play foods, not real foods. Most people who want to lose weight should not eat fruits. The fish-fowl-meats make the backbone of your diet, the real food.

Buying Fruits and Vegetables

First, it's important to buy *fresh* fruits and vegetables. Producers treat fruits and vegetables with chemicals before they can them, dry them, or freeze them. Don't bother to read the labels. The processors can legally add many chemicals without listing them on the label.

If possible, buy fruits and vegetables at farmers' markets. No matter what the farmer's wife tells you, don't expect her fruits and vegetables to be chemical free. Her produce, however, is likely to be purer than store-bought fruits and vegetables. Also, it's fresher.

You'll find some fruits and vegetables better at certain times of the year. After picking apples, for example, they treat them with God-only-knows-what chemicals and store them. At certain times of the year I can tolerate Yellow Delicious apples. At other times they make me tired and hungry. It depends upon how long they lay stored in their chemically blessed state.

Most fruits have been genetically selected so they are much sweeter than those found in nature. The entrepreneur farmer has learned that he can sell more fruits if they are sweet.

Most people are less reactive to fruit that's not quite ripe. Many of my patients can tolerate peaches or cantaloupes or other fruit if it's hard. When fully ripe, the sugar in fruits may addict you and send you on an eating spree.

Be careful about commercially bought grapes and berries. Many of them are moldy. Almost every person, overweight or not, has a body chemistry that is incompatible with mold.

When first starting the program, people should avoid grapes, pineapple, bananas, oranges and mangoes. They are often incompatible.

A few people can tolerate "organically" grown fruits and vegetables better than those grown commercially. They are worth a try, but they are not always the solution.

The Best Solution

1. Test fruits and vegetables to learn which you tolerate best.
2. Reduce your exposure to chemicals by eating no more than half a cup of vegetables three times a day.
3. Eat no more than one cup of fruit one to three times a day. If your weight stops melting away or if you find yourself getting hungry, omit all fruits.
4. Only eat fruits and vegetables with a fish-fowl-meat meal. The fat will slow down the speed with which fruits, vegetables and chemicals enter your body and reduce possible reactions.
5. Avoid beans (including bean sprouts) and root vegetables like carrots. Avoid all vegetables that you must cook before eating them.

Eat fruits and vegetables raw. (Didn't I promise you cooking wouldn't be a problem?) Why raw? It's been my clinical observation that patients who eat their fruits and vegetables raw gradually become less reactive. Cooking destroys something in foods. I don't know what. I simply know that I and my patients thrive better on raw foods.

In light of anthropology, that's not surprising. Although our ancestors have been using fire for 600,000 years, cooking did not become fashionable until the Würm ice age. The Würm glaciation lasted 65,000 years and ended about 12,000 years ago. Cooking is a Johnny-come-lately activity for mankind. Our body chemistry had many hundreds of millions of generations to adjust to uncooked foods.

Peel fruits and vegetables. I know that the peeling holds valuable nutrients. If you grow your own fruits and vegetables without the use of chemicals, then by all means eat the peelings. You should, however, peel commercially grown fruits and vegetables. They're all chemically contaminated. Farmers and manufacturers add more than 3,000 chemicals to the foods we eat. Even peeling doesn't avoid all the sprays, but it helps.

It's not possible to peel some fruits and vegetables—strawberries or celery, for example. Wash these with unscented soap and warm water. Rinse *well* before eating.

You should also peel or wash "organically grown" fruits and vegetables. Too often "organically grown" means only that they carry a high price tag.

Buying Fish-Fowl-Meat

Fish, fowl, and meat should be fresh, unaged, unpreserved. Do not buy canned, smoked foods or foods with nitrates in it.

You should select fatty fish: salmon, blue fish, black fish, mackerel, cod, shark and others. The fish you select should have bright eyes. If their eyes are dull, they have been in the shop too long. Susan Hecht, my assistant, says she looks in the fishes' eyes and only selects those which do not appear depressed!

Fish and chicken should have a firm feel to the flesh. It's a good idea to smell them before handing over your money. If you are too shy to smell them, pretend you're nearsighted. Squint your eyes and hold the chicken near your nose. Evolution had a reason for giving us a nose and for placing it just above our mouths!

Only about 40 percent of my patients can eat chicken without having an incompatible reaction. About 85 percent of my patients, however, can eat beef rib steaks without reacting. Which are you? You can only test and learn.

You may be able to eat one brand of chicken, but not another. I have two patients in Pennsylvania who can only eat chicken grown on their own farms. I had one patient who became tired after eating every brand of chicken she found in New York. She moved to Lexington, Kentucky. There, she could eat all the local brands.

As of this writing, the best-tolerated chicken in the New York area is fresh range-fed or fresh Kosher chicken. (Soak and wash kosher chicken well to remove the salt.) The next best is Holly Farms.

My patients do not react well to cut-up chicken parts. I suspect they paint antibiotics on cut-up chicken parts to keep them from spoiling.

Some people can tolerate the dark meat of chicken, but not the white meat and vice versa.

Always eat the skin on the chicken. You need the fat. One danger in eating chicken is that it may leave you hungry. You might cheat on your diet simply because you didn't have enough to eat. The fat will help satisfy you. (You may need to eat several chickens to feel satisfied!)

Some of my patients tolerate rock Cornish hens—even frozen ones—better than chickens.

Frozen duck is a big reactor. I've had no experience with fresh duck. Because the meat is fat, if tolerated, fresh duck and goose should be a good choice for weight losers.

Frozen turkeys are a bad trip for most of my patients. Many patients tolerate fresh turkey.

In general I feel that eating large amounts of chicken and other fowl is not the way to go. Commercial chickens are raised in such bizarre ways that I am not comfortable eating them.

If I had my own farm and raised my own chickens, I would feel much better about eating them. I would feel more comfortable eating ducks or geese that I raised and fed myself.

In general, I advise eating chicken, turkey, ducks and other fowl no more than once a week.

Fish

We've already talked about how to buy fish. You will recall that I advised fresh fatty fish. Eating dry (low-fat) fish leaves us hungry. Sooner or later people who eat dry fish will go off their diets and put on weight again.

I have one patient who reacts to all red meats. He thrives on fish. When he eats fish, he eats a plate piled high with fish and soaks it in butter. He has the lowest cholesterol on his block and not a pinch of fat on his body.

He likes cod liver oil so well he must be careful to keep from drinking too much. Linus Pauling tells me that when his son was little he had to watch the boy to make sure he didn't drink too much cod liver oil.

Fish is by far our most dangerous food. If you eat fish more than once a week, I would have it analyzed for heavy metals (such as mercury) and organic chemicals (such as PCBs) by the local health department. I would have it reanalyzed every two months.

Never eat raw or poorly cooked shellfish. The risk of hepatitis is too great. I would never eat *any* fish raw.

Airplanes and Delis

Almost everyone reacts to the preserved foods they serve on airlines. Take along your own food. Cook some beef rib steaks ahead of time, wrap them in aluminum foil and freeze them. Carry them with you in an insulated bag. Leave one steak out. In three or four hours it will defrost and be ready to eat.

Everything's wrong with deli foods. They sell preserved foods, frozen foods, seasoned foods, foods they cook with gas. The beef usually has little fat on it. For whatever reason, my patients have nothing but trouble with deli foods.

Buying Red Meats

Buy fresh, unaged beef. Steaks should be pink, not red. The meat should be moist and glistening. When shaken, the meat should flop about. Older steaks are red, dry, dull and tight.

People complain that unaged meat is tough. Be thankful. Your teeth, gums and jawbones need exercise like the rest of your body. If you don't exercise them, you will lose your teeth, your gums and the bone in your jaw.

Sorry, but you may also react to beef if it's *too* fresh. Meat should be at least three or four days old. If eaten raw, many patients tolerate very fresh meat. If the beef you buy is too fresh, wrap it in aluminum foil (dull side against the meat) and leave it in the refrigerator for two days to age. Then eat it or freeze it.

If the meat is more than a few days old, wrap it in foil and freeze it at once. *Before cooking, remove the foil. Do not use foil to catch the drippings.*

Do not buy dehydrated meat. It contains spices and preservatives. Many people do well on meat they dehydrate themselves. I've had good results with a dehydrator called Harvest Maid sold by Garden Way Catalog, Charlotte, Vermont 05445, 1-800-833-6990.

For dehydrating, use well-chilled meat with little fat on it. Round steak is usually a good choice. Slice it paper-thin. When you eat it, you will need to put butter or some fat on it. Some people do better on dehydrated rib steak. Only dehydrate the lean. Add some type of fat later when you eat it.

Dehydrated meat keeps well and is a very good solution for traveling. I have a patient who has a winter home in the center of Puerto Rico where it's impossible to buy good beef. She dehydrates her beef and takes along enough to last for two or three weeks.

Most of my patients do best eating mid-rib roasts cut into steaks. Do not, however, cook a rib roast and eat off it for several days—even refrigerated meat oxidizes. *Never, never reheat meat or fats*. Reheating oxidizes the fat. Oxidized fat may make you toxic or hungry. Also, it may give you cancer.

For years I have made the clinical observation that most patients feel best on marbleized fresh meat, such as beef rib steak. One of the reasons is that air does not reach and oxidize the central marbleized fat.

To reduce the surface of the fat exposed to the air, have the butcher cut steaks a least one and a quarter inches thick.

When buying red meats, have the butcher leave on the fat. After cooking the steak, trim off an eighth of an inch of fat and lean around the edges.

Steak like sirloin have no central fat, hence they are a poor choice. Most of my patients do not tolerate sirloin well. Different cuts of meat have different flavors. If they taste different, that means their chemistry is different.

The second-best tolerated type of beef is porterhouse steaks. People do well on filet mignon, but it has little fat on it.

To save money, some people eat chuck steak, veal or beef kidneys and hearts. They are usually well tolerated.

Cook with Electricity

In my view, no one should cook with gas, especially should we not cook fish, fowl and meats with gas. Twenty years ago when I became seriously interested in complex incompatibilities, I learned that many of my patients were incompatible with meats cooked in gas ovens. Those same patients could tolerate meats if cooked with electricity. The only conclusion: The fat in the meat absorbs gas.

Later I learned that all of my patients with asthma breathed markedly better after completely shutting off their gas stoves. This could only mean that gas escaped into the air and contributed to their attacks.

Reaction from gas may make people hungry. Also, remember that gas is a hydrocarbon. Hydrocarbons give people cancer. In my view, it should be illegal to allow gas into homes. Overweight people especially should avoid gas stoves.

An electrical stove is not practical for some people, especially those living in large apartment buildings. Recently one of my New York patients spent $20,000 to run a 220-volt line to her apartment.

I once owned a stove but gave it away. It's easy to cook with a counter-top broiler plus a one or two burner hot plate. One of the burners on the hot plate should be at least 750 watts. Most people are happier if one of the burners is 1000 watts.

No stove? Cook with a counter-top oven. Look, a microwave oven is nothing but a counter-top oven. Microwave ovens please many cooks.

My patients find toaster ovens quite satisfactory. I prefer a self-cleaning one like Toastmaster with an enamel rather than a plastic lining. Be sure to leave the door cracked open while broiling! Clean with hot water only. Clean only the pan and bottom.

Microwave Ovens

Don't rush out and buy a microwave oven. They present problems. Most people react better if the meat is left pink in the center. Microwaves quickly cook meat all the way through. Also, microwave ovens cook meat irregularly. They leave some of the meat raw, while overcooking other parts.

Aside from those reasons, my patients simply do not feel at their best when eating microwave-cooked meats. Exceptions: For some reason unknown to me, patients seem to tolerate fowl and pork chops equally well whether cooked in a broiler or in a microwave oven.

If you insist upon cooking with a microwave oven, to avoid radiation, stay an arm's length way from it. I have a patient whose daughter injured her hand by holding it over the microwave exhaust vent.

What is the long-term effect of eating microwave-cooked food? Ask me three generations from now and I'll give you a tentative answer.

Outdoor Grills

All grills overheat the surface of the meat. My patients do not do well on meat cooked on any grill. Especially they get reactions from meats cooked on outdoor charcoal or gas grills.

"That's the American way!" you protest.

Look, I only point out the facts. You must decide. Remember, if you live the all-American way, you'll die the all-American way: of complications from obesity, from diabetes, from a heart attack, stroke or cancer.

Convection Ovens

My patients don't do well on food cooked in convention ovens. Such ovens confine the heat. Super heating vaporizes fats. The fats penetrate the meat and it becomes toxic.

Open hearth broilers, like frying pans, overheat the surface of the meat and make it toxic. People have the same problem with broilers that have heating elements on two sides. They cook a steak on both sides at once and overheat it. The result: oxidized fat.

And if you have nothing but a counter-top toaster oven, count yourself lucky. It hasn't been that long since cooks built a fire in the yard and squatted over it—a one-burner fire—to cook the family meal.

Ventilation

One good thing about squatting over a fire to cook in the yard: The ventilation is excellent!

We must work out good ventilation for our kitchens. Many people stay overweight because they react to cooking fumes. I've seen many patients who reacted to gas fumes from kitchen stoves. Reactions have varied all the way from depression to headaches, to eating sprees. All cooking adds the odor of cooked food to the air. If you can smell it, then small particles of the food are floating in the air. When you breath these in, the body takes them in from the lungs. We can even react to fumes from broiling meat. The smoke particles that get into the air are particles of oxidized fat. You recall that oxidized fats are toxic.

The best ventilation is a hood and fan over the stove that vents fumes to the outside of the building. We must bring in fresh air to replace the vented air. Remember to leave the lower section of a window partly (at least 6 inches) open, either in the kitchen or in a nearby room.

As an alternative, buy a fan from the dime store that has extension panels. Mount the fan in the top section of the kitchen window. Have the fan push the air from inside to the outside. Leave the bottom section of the window cracked open.

Never bake your food. Baking, like cooking with a convection oven, confines, overheats and vaporizes fats so they not only become oxidized and toxic but actually penetrate the meat and thus ruin it.

Under ideal conditions, overweight people should not cook for anyone except themselves. If you must cook for the family, try to avoid cooking foods that contain grains, foods like spaghetti, bread and pies. Particles of the food get into the air, are breathed in and may knock out the turn-off cells in the appestat and send us on an eating spree.

Raw Fish, Fowl, Meats

Our body chemistry *cannot* use *raw* grains such as wheat. Our chemistry, however, can use raw fish, fowl, meats. I wouldn't advise eating raw fish or fowl, however, unless you know quite a bit about its origins. For example, I would want them grown in my own lake or on my own farm.

Pork, of course, must be cooked well to avoid trichinosis.

It's safer to eat raw lamb or beef if first it remains frozen for three days. Many of my patients, however, eat raw beef without freezing it first. None of them have experienced any difficulty from eating it raw.

People get all worked up when I speak of eating raw meat, yet steak tartare appears on the menu at many fine restaurants and steak tartare is ground raw beef. And consider this: if people eat their steaks or roast beef cooked rare or medium, the pink or red meat on the inside is nothing other than raw beef.

When you look at it that way, raw beef is really not a big deal.

A few of my patients are so reactive they can tolerate only raw meats. I saw such a patient the other day, a rabbi. He once said, "I don't know whether my synagogue would accept me if they knew I live on raw meat!"

Not long ago one of my patients who lives in London visited a butcher. The butcher mentioned that Nureyev, the ballet star, was a customer and ate raw meat. The other night one of my few raw-meat-eating patients visited me. There's nothing strange about the man. He's married, has several children and earns a living as a New York executive in one of America's largest and most conservative companies. He dare not go to work in anything other than a dark blue suit, white shirt and conservative tie.

He eats about 75 percent of his meat raw because he feels better on raw meat. This man first consulted me many years ago. Half a dozen physicians had treated him without realizing that he suffered from marked food incompatibilities. At the patient's first visit, he weighed 113 pounds and was about to starve. Today he weighs 157 pounds.

On the Newbold Diet, those who are underweight will gain, and those overweight will lose.

If you eat beef or lamb raw, you may cut it into small chunks, or grind it (as in steak tartare). Because ground meat ages rapidly, you should grind it just before eating it.

Some people will tolerate whole meat, but not tolerate the same meat if its ground. I'm not sure why. The reason may be that digestive juices act for a shorter time on ground meat. The meat breakdown products enter the body quickly.

Again let me remind you, whether you cook beef or eat it raw, do not eat the deckle on beef rib steaks. Rib steaks are usually well tolerated, but people often become ill when eating the deckle. The deckle is the tough outer part of a rib steak. Ask your butcher to identify it for you.

Cooking Meat, Fish, Fowl

You'll be happy to learn that most of my patients broil their fish, fowl and meats. Most people do best if they leave their beef, veal or lamb pink in the center.

A rare patient can avoid a reaction to meat only if it's cooked well.

Now and then I see a patient who can only eat meat cooked super-well in a pressure cooker.

People need to eat some of the white fat along with the lean meat. Throw away the browned or burned fat. Not only is the *burned and browned fat* a frequent cause of incompatibilities, it may give you cancer.

Boiling meat briefly gives the least oxidized meat and fat. Boiling is also the fastest and the least expensive way to cook. Most people react better if they leave the center of the meat pink. (Again, remember to cook pork well.)

Pan-frying is the most suspect way to cook meat. That's because the meat surface reaches a high temperature in a frying pan. If you eat pan-fried meat, fry it slowly so it doesn't burn.

The Big Secret

The trick to cooking is automation. My life style has always called for doing two or three things at once. It's not surprising that I learned how to cook and at the same time take a shower, or read, or write books.

My secret is an electric timer. The one I use *is not* a simple timer that rings to tell me when to turn my steak. My timer plugs into the wall electrical outlet. I then plug my hot plate or counter-top oven into the timer, set the timer and go about my business. When the time runs out, the oven will automatically cut off. At my leisure, I turn the steak and reset the timer. When finished cooking, the timer will again automatically cut off the oven or hot plate.

The timer I like has a 13-amp rating. I can set it for minutes. Most timers will not handle enough amps to use for ovens. Also, most of them time only 15-minute intervals. M. H. Rhodes, Inc. of Avon Connecticut, made the one that I use. You can also buy it at Rosetta Electric, 21 West 46th Street, New York, NY 10036.

Cleaning Up

Those of us who are reactive *should not use chemicals* to clean our ovens, cooking utensils, plates, flatware—or anything else. Hold the plate or fork under running hot water, scrub it with a metal brush, and dry it. If you feel compelled to scrub with something, use baking soda. Be sure to rinse thoroughly.

Restaurant Eating

More and more people in the well-off countries eat away from home. Dining out is often an important part of their social, business or family life. Restaurant eating, however, may present problems.

When you are first starting your diet, it's best to follow Carol Channing's method. One of my patients who is a friend of Miss Channing tells me that she's very food-reactive. She cooks a steak ahead of time, wraps it and places it in her purse. At the restaurant she orders something simple. When the food arrives, she smiles, pushes the food aside, takes her steak out of her purse and eats it.

"But I'm not Carol Channing. I can't pull that off," patients often tell me. Then order as best you can. Here are some tips.

Let's say that you do well on beef. Most restaurants have some form of beef or veal on the menu. You might try prime ribs. Tell the waiter that you *do not* want an end cut. Ask him not to pour any of the juices over your meat. The juice contains seasoning, oxidized fats, and many other things to which you will almost surely react. When your prime rib arrives, cut one-quarter inch of fat and meat from around the edge.

Trial and error will teach you that you may do better eating prime ribs at one restaurant than another.

Often steaks are available at restaurants, but most restaurants cook with gas. They broil steaks on an open gas grill. The fat on the meat will pick up hydrocarbons, exposing you to a reaction—and to cancer. You can get around this problem by asking them to pan-fry the steak at a low temperature in its own fat.

A cook in a small town such as Morning Sun, Iowa will respond to your request for a pan-fried steak, but you may have trouble in a city where cooks see themselves as artists and call themselves "chefs."

Recently I ordered a pan-fried steak in Mexico. The waiter said that they couldn't pan-fry a steak. My order resulted in a conference with half a dozen people, including the chef.

"We are absolutely unable to pan-fry a steak," the chef told me through a translator.

Finally, I said, "Can you fry an egg for me?"

"Oh, yes. No difficulty."

"Then take a steak, pretend it's an egg and fry it."

"But we don't fry steaks," he insisted.

"I would think," I said, "that you would get bored cooking the same way all the time. Wouldn't you like an exciting new adventure in cooking?"

No, he would not. He did not fry steaks!

I threw up my hands. In my room I ate the dehydrated beef chips I had brought along.

A number of chefs will respond favorably if you ask them to sauté your steak. They think "sauté" is high class, but "pan-frying" is low class. Of course *"sauté"* is only a French word that means "fry."

Often chefs have a block when you ask them to sauté a steak in its own fat. Sometimes it's best to ask them to sauté it in butter, which they also think is high class. Many reactive people can tolerate butter, especially in small amounts.

Many restaurants partially precook steaks and finish them off after the waiter brings in an order. Such a steak will have cross marks burned into it from the open grill. If you see cross marks, you know your steak wasn't sautéed. Send it back.

If the steak or veal chop is thick, ask them to butterfly it. Butterflying means splitting the meat in half to make it thinner. Chefs also think butterflying is high class and not beneath their artistic egoes. If they butterfly the meat, they're less likely to burn it. Tell them to cook it slowly. Warn them if they burn the steak, they'll only have to start all over again.

If they do burn the meat, cut a notch in it before they take it back. That prevents them from simply scraping it and returning the same piece of meat.

Many waiters don't listen to what patrons tell them. Most of their customers are semi-intoxicated by the time the meal arrives and don't know what they're eating.

Usually, you must tell a waiter everything three times. Then reach up and jerk the cuff of his sleeve and inform him that you're very reactive. If the restaurant doesn't follow your directions, they'll have to call an ambulance and cart you off to the emergency room.

Then add that your father is a world-famous trial lawyer. Tell him that the waiters, owners and chefs of the last three restaurants where you ate all had their property confiscated. Say that they're still in federal prisons in solitary confinement.

At this point, you may have the waiter's attention. Chances are he will ask, "What did you say?"

Maybe I've eaten too many times in New York restaurants. Also, I usually dress casually. Waiters glance at me, classify me as a patron with a thin purse and switch off their ears.

Try to be patient with the natives. Bear this in mind: After reading this book, you'll be living in the second half of the 21st century. The people around you are still struggling along in the second half of the 20th century.

In a restaurant you'll have less difficulty getting a fresh raw vegetable. Most of them have lettuce, celery or tomatoes.

Beware of fresh fruit in restaurants. The other day I had lunch with friends in a restaurant and virtuously ordered plain strawberries for dessert. They looked fresh and health-giving, but after eating them I turned drowsy.

Most restaurants cook with gas. Many have gas fumes in the dining area. When you first enter a restaurant, notice the atmosphere. If you sense gas, tell the maitre d' and retreat. In any case, don't let them sit you near the door that leads to the kitchen.

Be careful of restaurants that have picturesque candles burning on each table. Unless the air exchange is unusually good, the hydrocarbons from them may make you hungry. Restaurant owners love fat people!

Also be careful to avoid tobacco smoke and perfume. Remember, the world really is out to get you! You don't believe me? Look at the overweight people all around you. Something got them!

Truly, eating in a restaurant is a step in the dark.

14

Psychological Problems and Overweight

> *All our provisional ideas in psychology will someday be based on organic structure. This makes it probable that special substances and special chemicals control the operation.*
>
> —SIGMUND FREUD

Experience has taught me that psychological problems do not cause people to become overweight. Back in my Freud-oriented days, I thought that weight problems were basically psychological problems. My psychiatric colleagues and I talked about subconscious homosexual urges, Oedipus complexes, depression and anger. We even tried to cure weight problems with psychotherapy.

The simple truth is that psychological approaches sounded good, but never worked out. Psychotherapy did not help the patients lose weight.

Today I see overweight problems as essentially biochemical problems. That is not to say that overweight patients have no emotional problems. Commonly they suffer from emotional difficulties, *but their emotional symptoms are caused by the same food and environmental incompatibilities that make them overweight.*

As pointed out earlier, food intolerance can strike any organ in the body and cause that organ to malfunction. Intolerance to wheat can not only strike the *turn-off* cells in the appestat and send people on eating sprees, but may also strike the blood vessels and bring on hypertension, or may strike the knee joint and result in arthritis. So too an intolerance to wheat commonly reacts on the brain and causes emotional symptoms.

I have published articles on the subject in scientific journals and have written about it in various books. Others have made the same observations, especially F. C. Dohan at the University of Pennsylvania.

In this book I've already illustrated my thesis by telling how milk gave Mary Lou Masterson emotional symptoms. Food incompatibilities gave Don Sordi the comedian some of his emotional symptoms. I mentioned the "Christmas neurosis" brought on by excessive intake of carbohydrates that are incompatible with many biochemistries.

But When I Get Upset, I Eat

True, people often eat when they feel tension, anger or depression. That doesn't mean that the emotional upheaval caused the eating spree.

Here's what happens: *The same incompatibility (from things like wheat, sugar or milk or fumes from a photostat machine or gas from the kitchen stove) that strikes our brains and gives us emotional symptoms also strikes the turn-off cells in our appestats and makes us hungry.*

JOAN BAKER

Joan was a 48-year-old, well-educated white married woman who weighed 243 pounds. Because Joan was six feet tall, some people might call her a big woman rather than a fat woman. I looked upon her as a big, fat woman. She wore a dark, aggressive expression on her face. Hers was a face you would expect to see beneath a tabloid headline telling how she had axed her husband to death for failing to make her morning coffee.

For four years she had wandered in and out of my office trying to lose weight. She would start on a weight reduction program, follow it for three or four weeks, then disappear for six months or a year.

Because of incompatibilities, wheat and sugar made Joan not only overweight but also extremely angry. From previous contacts with her, I had observed that her thought processes and behavior were relaxed and pleasant when all wheat and sugar was removed from her diet.

Because Joan was unwilling to stop eating wheat and sugar and break her addiction to them, she remained overweight. Incompatibility with wheat and sugar also kept her chronically angry.

"This is an emergency!" she told me one afternoon on the telephone. "I absolutely must see you right away." When she rushed into my office, she said, "I've gone wild! You've got to help me!"

She had found herself about to be late for her appointment with me. She risked her life by running through the rush-hour streets of Manhattan frantically searching for a taxi.

Working with Joan had taught me that Joan had come to enjoy exposing herself to danger. Excitement discharged her anger and left her feeling relaxed.

During her appointment, Joan informed me that she once again had fallen "madly in love" with a "very intelligent" but uneducated 21-year-old man named Coke. Previously she had told me about similar romances. Coke, like her other lovers, was sex-starved, penniless, and fresh from prison. This lover had been in prison for shooting a guard during a holdup.

After two hours of violent sex, during which her ex-con lover would pull her ears, belt her around and almost kill her, Joan would feel completely free of anger. The sexually oriented excitement and danger temporarily discharged her anger and for a time left her feeling as peaceful as an angel singing in a church choir.

She gave the fresh-from-prison young man sex and money. No amount of sex and money, however, could hold the violent, unstable young man for more than a few weeks. Shortly before Joan saw me, Coke had "fallen in love" with a woman his own age. While making love to Joan, Coke told her details about his passionate coupling with the other woman.

A Psychological Problem?

Most psychiatrists and psychologists would say that Joan had an emotional problem that she needed to work out.

I strongly disagree. Most mental health professionals would not even suspect the real cause of her emotional upheaval was food incompatibilities.

After her visit with me, Joan went on her diet again. She gave up wheat and sugar. As before, she not only lost weight, but also lost her anger and her need for danger.

"I've started eating just a small amount of wheat again," she remarked as she was leaving my office one day.

"You can't control it," I reminded her, concerned. "You're like an alcoholic, only with you it's wheat and sugar."

As before, she would not listen to reason. Joan is proof that addictions are among the strongest forces in the universe, stronger than love and honor, often stronger even than the desire to live.

As before, she gradually got off her diet. Her seething anger returned, and she became angry with me. When she consulted a psychologist, he told her that her problems were psychological and that she could eat all the wheat and sugar she desired. She left me to be treated by the psychologist.

About a year later the six o'clock news showed Joan's half-covered body lying in a pool of blood in a motel room. She was no longer angry. The pushers—the wheat and sugar pushers—had won again.

MIRIAM STEIN

Miriam Stein was a 190-pound, 51-year-old woman who suffered from obesity and depression. She wore black clothes and had a head full of black thoughts. Like many depressed people, she suffered from chronic fatigue. In my office she sat and sighed as she told me that she could not lose weight and could not get her life together.

Miriam, whose husband was a well-off stockbroker, had spent the last several years trying to turn her apartment into the castle of her dreams. She had the workmen put up walls, then tear them down. They mounted cabinets in her kitchen. She decided they weren't quite right and replaced them. She watched them hang wallpaper, changed her mind, then changed it again. For nearly two years she had constantly lived with dust, fresh paint and new carpeting.

Gradually, she stopped going out to lunch with her friends. She sat at home and nibbled on chocolates as she supervised the workmen. She grew fat and depressed.

Empty nest syndrome? True, her children had left. They no longer needed her to take them to school or to sit up with them at night when they had the croup. Nevertheless, her weight was normal and she was getting along well enough until she started creating her dream castle.

Miriam had surrounded herself with chemicals (wallpaper, wallpaper glue, paint, varnish, etc.) which were incompatible with her body chemistry.

Her imcompatibility with the chemicals knocked out the *turn-off* cells in her appestat center and gave her a *Type-A* overweight problem. She spree-ate. Her sprees were not dramatic. She had no chasing-around-town-for-food eating sprees. She had one long eating spree that lasted all day, every day. She simply nibbled away at chocolate.

I suspected that she had also developed an addiction to the chocolates and also suffered from a *Type-B* overweight problem.

How did I know what was happening without first testing her? I knew from listening to her history. A detailed history is the most important diagnostic tool ever discovered by man. Unfortunately, because a careful history is time-consuming, it's badly neglected by the medical profession. Also, patients aren't mesmerized by a careful history. They are more impressed by the inferior multimillion-dollar MRI machine they've been told about on TV news programs. MRI machines are good show biz. Sick people have always preferred the medicine man who puts on a good show before selling them a bottle of snake oil.

Unfortunately, American medicine is being corrupted by the insurance industry, which is run by clerks and computers. They understand paying out $200 for a proctoscopic examination that takes 10 minutes to perform. For a worthwhile history that takes the doctor an hour, they pay $30 for a routine office visit. Do you understand why most doctors do procedures, but neglect histories? Do you see how the patient suffers from clerk-and-computer medicine? The price of medicine is certainly going up, but not the quality.

How did I know that Miriam was suffering weight problems because of incompatibilities? I knew because I had seen so many other patients with similar symptoms caused by similar incompatibilities. How do you know your mother when you see her? She looks like your mother, she walks like your mother, she talks like your mother. You don't need to do an MRI scan, a biopsy and X-ray examinations of her teeth to identify her.

In an attempt to work out this patient's incompatibilities, I asked her to bring in photographs of her apartment. I had never seen such confusion: piles of lumber everywhere, Sheetrock stacked here and there, half-used buckets of paint. The place was an absolute disaster for a chemically sensitive person.

I asked her to start by keeping some windows open to at least dilute the fumes.

She didn't want to open the windows. She had grown to like the draperies drawn and the windows closed!

I asked her to get out of the apartment and take walks in the park.

She had to stay and watch the workmen!

I asked her to change her diet and take nutritional supplements.

She tried to, but the chemicals in her apartment left her brain so confused that she couldn't get organized well enough to either cook her food or take the vitamins and other supplements I recommended.

Was she depressed? Yes, but her depression came from chronic exposure to chemicals in her home. Moreover, she has a brain chemistry incompatible with chocolate and sugar. Her poor diet gave her vitamin and mineral deficiencies, which further worsened both her body chemistry and her brain chemistry.

She was depressed, but psychology had nothing to do with her depression or her obesity. *Chemical* insults—not *psychological* insults—made her depressed.

She would remain depressed and overweight until she removed the incompatible chemicals from her home and stopped eating foods that gave her incompatibility reactions. Of course, she also needed extra vitamins and minerals.

We made absolutely no progress with this patient until her husband, at my recommendation, employed a housekeeper, closed the apartment and moved the patient to their summer home on Long Island. Once away from the multiple chemicals contaminating her apartment, she rapidly lost weight. Her depression lifted. Twice she returned to her apartment in the city for brief periods. Both times, within an hour, her depression returned and along with it her desire for chocolate.

Now I Lay Me Down to Sleep

Do you remember this childhood prayer? We all know there is something special about the night. Night is a mystery, a time when we lose control. We travel into the land of the ghosts of time past and the not quite fully realized loves of our lives as well as a threatening place where the spirits of our enemies sometimes threaten us.

At night our primitive fears and pleasures come out and roam about. We leave behind the conscious world. We no longer have our intellect or our sense of sight and smell to protect us from shadowy threats. We are born with a fear of the night, of the dark mysteries that live in the other world that we long to visit but cannot control.

Poets have called sleep "the little death."

When we fall asleep at night, we all fear that we will not wake up in the morning. We worry about not returning to the world of sunlight where we have learned to make our way in relative safety.

People mate for many reasons. Among the more important reasons is to have a companion to sleep with at night. I speak of literal sleep, not the act of lovemaking. However pleasant sex might be, it's even more pleasant to have someone we love and trust to sleep with us at night. We like someone we trust with us when we enter the dangerous land of dark mysteries.

Sleeping together is a much more intimate relationship than having sex together. When we have sex, we are at least more or less conscious and in control of events. When we sleep, we lower our defenses and become helpless. We need to be with someone we know will not take our money or plunge a knife through our heart.

Nighttime Eating

Because we all fear the night, eating at night takes on a special meaning. Many people have a weight problem because their eating gets out of control at night.

Depressed people halfway want to die—yet down deep they mostly want to live. Because of their need to die, depressed people especially fear the night. People often drink milk or eat sweets because these make them sleepy. *They mistake toxicity for relaxation.*

We have an expression: "I ate myself into a coma."

Using toxicity to go to sleep is about as logical as hitting yourself in the head with a hammer to bring on sleep.

Some night eaters are trying to avoid withdrawal reactions. As you have already learned, withdrawal from a food to which you have an incompatibility will usually make you tense and restless.

Others drink alcoholic beverages at night to put themselves to sleep.

If you put yourself to sleep with foods or beverages to which are incompatible with your chemistry, chances are several things will happen:

1. You will have bad dreams.
2. You will awaken tired.
3. You will feel depressed when you wake up.
4. You will wake up in the middle of the night and not be able to fall back asleep.
5. You will wake up early in the morning.
6. *You will become overweight.*

Night eating is not the way to go. Night eaters are using foods that are toxic (incompatible) as sedatives.

When you come off the foods to which you are addicted, be prepared to sleep poorly for three nights. Then you will sleep better than ever before.

Insomnia is not a sign of intelligence. It's a sign of cerebral food incompatibilities. Few physicians know this.

Many wealthy and powerful men (including Artistotle Onassis) suffered all their lives from hellish insomnia simply because of undiagnosed untreated incompatibilities with food and drink.

In Summary

If we straighten out our *chemical* problems, our *psychological* problems fall into place. We need to go on the proper vitamins and minerals. We must clean up our environment. Above all, we must stay away from food and drink that is incompatible with our particular chemistry. Then we can forget about emotions. Like breathing, emotions will take care of themselves.

15

Anorexia, Bulimia and Emesis (Loss of Appetite, Excessive Hunger and Throwing Up)

*Was this the face that launched a thousand ships,
And burned the topless towers of Ilium?*

—CHRISTOPHER MARLOW

DORIS WELCH

This tall, slender, charming 25-year-old blonde looked like a Viking princess. She had style and came across as a bright woman completely in charge of herself and everything around her.

Doris was from a well-off family with an apartment on Fifth Avenue and an estate on Long Island. She graduated *cum laude* from Smith and now held an executive position in one of New York's more competitive industries. If you talked with this seemingly totally together young woman at a cocktail party or consulted her about a business matter, you would think that she might one day have a shot at becoming the president of NBC or IBM.

Doris, however, suffered from *bulimia*. Almost every night she would go on an ice-cream-and-chocolate-cake binge. After gorging herself, she would shove two fingers down her throat and force herself to throw up. If you looked closely, you would notice that she had calluses on the backs of her second and third fingers. The calluses came from pushing her fingers past her front teeth as she stuck her fingers down her throat.

As you might suspect, tests proved that wheat, sugar and chocolate were incompatible with her chemistry. They knocked out the *turn-off* cells in her appestat. Although slender, Doris suffered from a *Type-A* (spree eating) weight problem. She controlled her weight by throwing up.

Doris had another reason to bring on vomiting. If she didn't throw up immediately after her eating spree, she became angry and depressed.

She was in love with a Wall Street broker. If she failed to throw up directly after spree-eating, she would become angry with her boyfriend. She would pick fights with him. They were no ordinary fights. She would end up screaming and trying to belittle him.

Whenever he mentioned her bouts of vomiting, she passed them off as "something I ate." Instead of going to the bathroom where he could hear her throw up, she began locking herself in the bedroom closet at the end of the hall and using plastic bags. She hid them in her closet. After discovering the bags, it began to dawn on her stunned boyfriend that this seemingly together woman had a major problem.

Finally, after she continued to refuse professional help, he left her. Only then did she consult me.

"He said that being with me did a number on his head," she told me through tears.

It took Doris about three months to come to grips with my program. She would eat only the foods that were compatible with her chemistry for five or six days. Then she would have a drink or two and say to hell with Dr. Newbold and the diet. Once again she would spree-eat and throw up.

Finally, I convinced her to stop drinking. That was the turning point. As long as she had no alcoholic beverages, she could avoid the foods that were not compatible with her chemistry.

Not only did she remain slender, but quickly she lost all interest in spree eating and throwing up. Having avoided the cause of her anger, anger was no longer a problem. She began settling down with a new boyfriend.

Bulimia

The dictionary tells us that bulimia is an "abnormal and constant craving for food." In our society it has come to mean spree eating followed by throwing up.

The ancient Greeks knew about bulimia. During classical times, wealthy Romans popularized it. Later, in 1937, I first learned about the condition. My girlfriend's older sister mentioned that she had eaten too much at lunch and retreated to the powder room to "fountain face."

Bulimia and anoxrexia are disorders associated with civilization and wealth. Mankind solves one problem only to create a new one.

The medical profession shows little interest in bulimia. I recently checked several textbooks widely used by physicians and found not a single word about it. Perhaps part of this neglect is because physicians are unable to treat bulimia successfully. In general, the medical profession does not understand food and enviromental incompatibilities.

As usual, when the profession does not understand an illness, it tosses it into that great wastebasket labeled "psychiatric."

Bulimia has become a common disorder in our society. Ninety-five percent of the time it occurs in young women. I've always treated it as nothing other than another food or environmental incompatibility. Its treatment is the same as for hives or migraine headaches.

A few bulimia patients refuse to test certain foods such as beef. I have nothing to offer such patients.

The cooperative patients all recover. Whether slowly or rapidly depends upon how soon they begin to follow directions. They must learn how to avoid foods that knock out their *turn-off* cells.

People suffering from bulimia may also have environmental incompatibilities. Some of them will not recover unless they give away their cats, cut off their gas stoves, stop smoking, use unscented makeup, sleep on all-cotton pillows, etc.

Anorexia

Anorexia means prolonged loss of appetite. It can come from many serious diseases. For example, the patient with tuberculosis or malaria and a temperature of 103 will lose his appetite and suffer from anorexia.

When treating such medical diseases, physicians concentrate on curing the underlying trouble. They know that once the underlying disease is cured, patients will lose their anorexia and start eating again.

Unfortunately, back in 1873 the medical profession labeled anorexia "anorexia nervosa." Since then, when patients suffer from anorexia without any recognizable medical disease like typhoid fever, the profession assumes that anorexia is emotional in origin. It's the same old mistake the profession has been making for more than a hundred years. If physicians do not know the cause of a disorder, they label it "neurotic" and forget about it.

Many disorders labeled neurotic or psychotic are due either to food or environmental incompatibilities, or to nutritional deficiencies.

If people suffering from anorexia are placed on foods that are compatible with their particular body chemistry and are given proper amounts of vitamins, minerals and unsaturated fats, they will quickly recover.

BARBARA HUTTON

Your mothers and fathers will remember Barbara Hutton (1912–1979) as the "poor little rich girl" who inherited the Woolworth dime-store fortune. From investments she had an income of two million dollars a year back during the depression of the 1930s. In those days a nickle would buy a bottle of Coca-Cola.

Barbara apparently suffered from food incompatibilities that gave her both *type-A* and *type-B* weight problems. Incompatibilities explain her weight problem and the bulimia and anorexia that followed.

After her first wedding (the first of seven), Barbara Hutton and her husband were on a night train hurtling through the darkness on the way from Paris to Lake Como. When she undressed and started to put on a designer silk-and-lace nightgown, her brand-new husband said, "Barbara, you're too fat!"

She was five-feet, 4-inches tall and weighed 148 pounds.

She never got over his remark. She didn't, however, remain "fat" much longer. She became bulimic and anorexic for the remainder of her life.

During a birthday celebration, a biographer reports that Barbara had one of her rare meals: cheeseburgers, French fries and Coca-Cola. She then locked herself in the lavatory and threw up. One of her typical dinners was a dozen bottles of Coca-Cola and one bottle of fresh milk.

Although doctors gave her vitamin injections, she must have been very deficient in saturated and unsaturated fats, minerals and proteins. Because she felt so miserable, she became addicted to alcohol and multiple drugs.

Food incompatibilities were behind many of her problems, which included:

1. Psychopathic personality.
2. Paranoia.
3. Chronic depression.
4. Multiple addictions (cigarettes, alcohol, drugs).
5. Multiple fractures.
6. Weakness.
7. Loss of teeth.
8. Bulimia.
9. Anorexia.
10. Heart failure and death.

It's easy to understand why deficiencies develop when people eat like Barbara Hutton. Deficiencies join incompatibilities to injure the cells in the appestat. When the *turn-on* cells begin to fail, nothing tells the person to eat. The result: anorexia.

The Mirror Says I'm Fat!

People with bulimia worry about their weight. They insist that they are overweight when they appear thin to everyone else. You cannot shake that belief. Psychiatrists say that bulimic patients have delusions about their body weight.

The patients know more about their conditions than the doctors. They know that they cannot control their spree eating. They have learned that they can gain weight rapidly. I once had a physician's wife as a patient who could eat one saucer of ice cream and gain 15 pounds. Her body chemistry was incompatible with ice cream. Like some patients with incompatibilities, she stored water in her tissues whenever she ate an incompatible food.

If anorexic patients see themselves as being overweight when others do not, it's because they know how quickly their bodies can balloon to elephantine sizes.

That is the interesting aspect of the Newbold Diet. Those who are underweight gain on it; those who are overweight, lose weight.

Warning

Bulimia and anorexia are not minor problems. As with Barbara Hutton, they can ruin the quality of life and lead to death. Everyone with these disorders should seek the professional care of a physician well-versed in treating food and environmental incompatibilities.

Some patients might get better after prolonged work with "counselors" and the average allergist and psychistrist, but they are patients who would have gotten better anyway. Usually those who improve with counseling and psychiatric care remain more or less crippled in one way or another and fail to reach their potentials in life.

Several years ago I saw a young woman who had been unsuccessfully treated at a famous and very expensive psychiatric hospital. My testing revealed that she had a disastrously low vitamin B12 level. The center had been so sure that her trouble was psychological that they hadn't bothered to test her B12 level. With a low B12 there was no way they could possibly help her.

Anorexia and bulimia are biochemical problems and can only be successfully cured by biochemical approaches. Once the biochemistry is taken care of, everything else will fall into place. Allergists have nothing to offer these patients.

16

Tranquilizers, Antidepressants and Weight Loss

Man's nature, like his body, is a product of evolution.
—ROBERT ARDREY

Female Sex Hormones

Ruth weighed 197 pounds when she first visited my office. Now, three months later, she has lost only 15 pounds. She should have lost 24 to 36 pounds.

On her first visit, I told her, "If you stay on your birth control pills, you'll have trouble taking weight off."

She didn't care. Life without her birth control pills wasn't worthwhile. She hated an IUD and found a diaphragm unromantic. Her boyfriend didn't like condoms.

She's winning her weight battle, but slowly, too slowly for my taste. I like to see patients lose two to three pounds a week. That's 50 to 75 pounds in six months.

It's the same with menopausal women who take hormones. Losing weight isn't easy.

Parenthetically, here's good news for women who take female sex hormones to avoid hot flashes. If you stay away from foods and other things that are incompatible with your chemistry, hot flashes almost always fade away. If a few remain, vitamin E will usually banish them.

142

Male Sex Hormones

Ted Jackson consulted me a few months ago because he wanted to lose 15 pounds. During the initial interview, I learned he was taking testosterone (a male sex hormone) injections once a week for impotency. It's also difficult for men to lose weight when they take male sex hormones.

Now and then you hear comments on TV about weight lifters, professional football players and other athletes using steroids to improve their muscle mass, their appearance and their performance. You can bet that they don't take the hormones to *lose* weight.

"Getting weight off and keeping it off will be difficult," I told Ted. "In spite of the hormone injections, you can lose weight, but you won't lose if you cheat on your diet even now and then."

Ted had a problem. He enjoyed a drink or two with sex. Then, after a drink or two and an hour of sex, he liked to top off his evening with a couple of slices of cheesecake. He saw me for six weeks. He would lose a pound, then gain a pound. Up and down, around and around he went with his weight loss program.

"Especially can you not take hormones, cheat and lose weight," I reminded him.

Finally, he took off 10 pounds, then it was the same old up one week and down the next.

"You've got to make a choice," I finally told him. "What do you want?"

Like all of us, Ted wanted to have his cake and eat it too. He can't win. He's trying to play games with Mother Nature. She doesn't give any points for nice smiles and firm handshakes. Either you follow her rules and win, or you don't follow her rules and fail.

Americans seem to view firm rules as unfair. They often act as if they think Mother Nature should make exceptions for them just because they live in the Land of the Free and the Home of the Brave. Believe me, Mother Nature couldn't care less. We do things Her way, or we don't get what we want from Her.

Finally, Ted said he'd had enough. He wanted his booze and his cheesecake and his hormone shots and he would forget about his bulging waist line.

We all have to make choices. If we have a weight problem and choose to take sex hormones and want to keep our weight normal, we must toe the dietary line 365¼ days a year.

Thyroid Hormones and Weight Loss

I seldom prescribe thyroid, but I have had many years experience with it. Some people lose weight better when taking thyroid hormones. This is especially true if patients have dry skin and hair, and often feel chilly when other people feel comfortable. The traditional view is that people lose weight better if they take thyroid hormones because it helps them "burn their food faster." I have clinical evidence that taking thyroid hormones reduces incompatibilities. I suspect that's the main reason people often lose weight better when taking thyroid hormones.

Taking any hormone is not a do-it-yourself project. If you use them, you must be under the care of a physician. The physician should not, however, make the common mistake of prescribing the hormone only if blood tests show a deficiency. The longer I'm in practice, the more firmly I believe that a therapeutic trial is the most valuable test for thyroid deficiency. *Therapeutic trial* means giving a medication and observing whether a patient feels better or worse on it.

I order blood tests on all of my new patients to measure thyroid hormones. Sometimes, however, I give thyroid hormones to patients and observe whether the patient feels better or worse. A. J. Prange Jr. at the University of North Carolina has advocated giving thyroid to all depressed patients even if tests fail to show they are low in the hormone. His successes prove him right.

If more physicians read E. R. Pickney's article in the *Archives of Internal Medicine* they would have less faith in laboratory tests. Ultimately, only the body can tell us if we need more thyroid hormone.

Broda Barnes, M.D., Ph.D., probably knows more about thyroid than anyone. He spent his professional life prescribing whole thyroid, Armour brand. Why? He finds that whole beef thyroid acts more like human thyroid than any other. Also, it's his observation that patients do better on whole beef thyroid.

Why Armour brand? Figures comparing the standardization of Armour thyroid tablets with other brands show that the Armour assays are more accurate than the others. (Anyone who thinks a generic medication is always as good as a brand-name medication has not worked closely enough with patients to learn the facts.)

If you ask many of the "modern" physicians why they prescribe synthetic thyroid hormone rather than the natural, they'll tell you that the natural is not standardized well enough. Most of them don't know. They've never used it. They got their information out of a book written by a physician who copied the information from another book written by a doctor who also had no experience with the product.

I've tried various types of thyroid. I know firsthand what works and what doesn't work. Follow my advice: Ask your physician to try you on Armour brand thyroid first. If it doesn't work out, then go to one of the synthetics.

The biggest problem with Armour thyroid is that it has traces of iodine. If acne bothers you, it's often better to use one of the synthetic hormones.

Then there are the few patients out of every hundred who do better on one of the synthetic thyroid hormones. Why? I don't know. Each of us has a unique chemistry.

When I come across a rare patient who does not tolerate Armour thyroid, my next choice is Synthroid.

Many physicians make the mistake of starting patients on doses of thyroid that are too large. When I use it, I start patients on Armour thyroid, 30 mg after breakfast and build it up slowly. I seldom go beyond 60 to 120 mg daily. This type of thyroid helps some people right away. Others take up to two months to show full effect.

Cortical Steroids

Steroids like prednisone given for diseases such as arthritis and asthma are a serious problem for all patients, especially for patients who want to lose weight. Adrenal cortical hormones make bones lose calcium, give moonshaped faces, and too often drive people out of their heads.

Losing weight while on more than 5 mg a day of prednisone is even more difficult than when taking sex hormones. The good news is, if people avoid the foods and environmental things which are incompatible with their body chemistry, they hardly ever need adrenal cortical steroids such as prednisone.

Major Tranquilizers and Antidepressants

What are tranquilizers and antidepressants doing in a chapter on hormones?

Just this: the major tranquilizers, like Thorazine, knock out the appetite centers and make most people gain weight. The same is true for antidepressants. You can lose weight while taking them, but as with hormones, weight loss is difficult and there's absolutely no room for cheating.

The good news is, when you eat the right diet, you almost surely will not need the tranquilizers and/or antidepressants.

17

Losing Weight and Lowering Your Cholesterol While Eating a High Animal Fat Diet

A high level of vitamin C increases the amount of high-density and decreases the amount of low-density lipoprotein cholesterol. Both of these changes help to protect against cardiovascular disease.

—LINUS PAULING

Weight losers, TV commercials and members of the American Heart Association have called animal fat the world's arch villain.

I have learned that *animal fat can be a hero in disguise—if you learn the rules for eating it.*

Animal fat interests me because:

1. Many people find animal fat more compatible with their body chemistry than carbohydrates such as grains, sugar, milk, beans, and nuts.
2. Eating animal fats is the easiest, surest way to lose weight.

My Cholesterol

As you may recall, 20 years ago I discovered that my cholesterol was a dangerous 312.

To my utter surprise, on a high red meat, high animal fat diet my cholesterol level *fell* from 312 to under 200. I was surprised again two

147

weeks ago when I had my cholesterol tested again—for the first time in 10 years—and discovered it was 132!

I have learned that I (as well as my patients) can eat fatty rib steaks three times a day and still have a low cholesterol. It helps to take certain vitamins, minerals and unsaturated fats. Also, we need to leave sugar, grains, milk products, beans and nuts *totally* out of our diets.

Most of the patients who consult me do not have a high cholesterol level. Those who have a low cholesterol keep their cholesterol low on a high animal fat diet. For example, I have a patient in Miami who was so sensitive that she could hardly eat anything other than beef rib steaks. She ate that way for 10 years. Her cholesterol was 180 when she first visited me. For years I didn't bother to recheck her cholesterol. Because she had no choice but to eat the rib steak diet, it made no difference what her cholesterol might be. If we found it high, it would only disturb her.

Then I began to observe other patients lowering their cholesterol levels while eating diets high in animal fat and, out of curiosity, rechecked her cholesterol level. Her cholesterol had been 180 when she started the high animal fat diet. It was still, after 10 years of eating mostly fatty beef rib steak, 180!

Several years ago I collected seven patients who at the time of their first visit had elevated cholesterol levels. I gathered the facts about these patients and published the findings in two respected, peer-reviewed, Index Medicus-listed medical journals. A short version appeared in the *International Journal for Vitamin and Nutrition Research* and a longer version was in the *Southern Medical Journal.*

Experience with more patients since then has supported my original findings.

High Density Lipoproteins (HDL)

To understand cholesterol, you need to know about HDL. HDL stands for high density lipoproteins. HDL is the "good" fat. You want it high. The American Heart Association, and everyone else, agrees that the higher the HDL, the less chance you have of suffering a stroke or heart attack. Authorities agree that HDL levels are more important than cholesterol levels in predicting who will have a heart attack or stroke, and who will not.

HDL percentage is a weighted HDL figure that shows the relationship between HDL and cholesterol. The higher the HDL percentage, the better. The HDL percentage is more meaningful than the simple HDL figure.

Triglycerides

Triglycerides are another group of fats in the bloodstream. High triglyceride levels are accompanied by an increased incidence of strokes and heart attacks. Most commonly high triglyceride levels are associated with a diet high in carbohydrates. Among my patients, triglyceride levels almost always fall, as they did in the patients you will soon meet. Low triglyceride levels are desirable.

Patients

When the patients discussed below first visited me, they were eating ordinary, varied American diets, but were suffering from various manifestations of food incompatibilities.

Elimination food tests revealed that each of these patients could best tolerate beef rib steaks. For varying times these patients ate mostly unaged beef rib steaks. Some were able to tolerate lamb, pork, or chicken if eaten no more than once every three or four days. Those patients occasionally ate pork, lamb or chicken in place of the rib steak. Rarely they ate cuts of beef other than rib steaks.

Patients asked their butchers to leave a large percentage of the fat on the steaks. To satisfy their hunger, patients ate as much of the fat as they could comfortably handle.

The only other foods they ate were up to one cup of fresh raw vegetables one to three times a day, and up to one cup of fresh raw fruit one to three times a day. They used no seasoning. They drank only bottled spring water (or self-distilled water), at least one-and-a-half quarts daily. The patients also took vitamins, minerals, and used polyunsaturated fats.

Each patient cooked the food with electricity and ate none of the deckle. They ate no browned or burned fat. All of their beef was unaged.

They peeled fruits and vegetables where possible. Otherwise, they washed them.

Test Before and After High Animal Fat Diets

All tests were performed after an overnight fast. Laboratory tests were *not* performed in my office, but at various state-approved and cerified clinical laboratories.

Patient One, 35-year-old white male.

FIRST VISIT:		NINE MONTHS LATER:	
cholesterol	278	cholesterol	188
triglycerides	165	triglycerides	69
HDL	35	HDL	58
% HDL	13	% HDL	30
glucose	118	glucose	93

Patient Two, a 48-year-old white male.

FIRST VISIT:		SIX MONTHS LATER:	
cholesterol	298	cholesterol	191
triglycerides	149	triglycerides	87
HDL	57	HDL	65
% HDL	19	% HDL	34

Patient Three, a 56-year-old white male. At his first visit he was on oral medication in an attempt to reduce his blood sugar. He stopped the medication after two weeks under my supervision.

FIRST VISIT:		AFTER 12 WEEKS:	
cholesterol	234	cholesterol	166
triglycerides	102	triglycerides	75
HDL	40	HDL	32
% HDL	17	% HDL	19
blood sugar	216	blood sugar	98

Patient Four, a 58-year-old white female.

FIRST VISIT:

cholesterol	327
triglycerides	65
HDL	90
% HDL	28

ONE-AND-A-HALF YEARS LATER:

cholesterol	209
triglycerides	58
HDL	87
% HDL	42

Patient Five, a 60-year-old white male.

FIRST VISIT:

cholesterol	224
triglycerides	128
HDL	47
% HDL	21

FOUR MONTHS LATER:

cholesterol	168
triglycerides	84
HDL	42
% HDL	25

Patient Six, a 63-year-old white male. At the time of his first visit he was eating a "low-cholesterol diet" that included lean red meat only once a week.

FIRST VISIT:

cholesterol	252
triglycerides	92
HDL	74
% HDL	29

THREE MONTHS LATER:

cholesterol	220
triglycerides	75
HDL	92
% HDL	42

Patient Seven, a 72-year-old black male.

FIRST VISIT:

cholesterol	228
triglycerides	90
HDL	100
% HDL	42

FIVE MONTHS LATER:

cholesterol	183
triglycerides	68
HDL not repeated	

Results

As you can see, *before starting a high animal fat diet, these patients had an average serum cholesterol of 263. Their average serum cholesterol levels fell to 189.*

At the same time their *triglycerides fell from an average of 113 to 74.*

One of the patients did not have a repeat HDL test. In the six patients retested for HDL, the *HDL percentages rose from 21 to 32.*

Only two of the patients were overweight (Patient One and Patient Three). They had a significant weight loss.

I have had many more patients show similar changes since.

Not Alone

A.B. Nichols and his fellow workers reported in the *Journal of the American Medical Association* in 1976 on 4,057 citizens studied in the town of Tecumseh, Michigan. The report concluded that *what the people ate had no relationship to their cholesterol levels.*

Only their weight correlated with their cholesterol levels. Those people who were overweight had higher cholesterol levels.

Several years ago the *Journal of the American Medical Association* published another study on cholesterol that *said that with at least two thirds of the population, what they ate had no bearing on their cholesterol levels.*

The article implied that the food industry had latched onto a good thing and was trying to take advantage of the American public by building false hopes about what food could do to lower cholesterol levels.

The late Roger Williams, Ph.D. was the Professor of Biochemistry at the University of Texas, Director of Clayton Foundation Biochemical Institute, University of Texas, formerly president of the American Chemical Society, discoverer of the B vitamin pantothenic acid, pioneer in folic acid research, gave folic acid its name. No one ever called him an irresponsible reporter. In his internationally respected book, *Nutrition Against Disease*, Roger Williams has this to say about cholesterol:

> How can this deposit of cholesterol be prevented? The most obvi-
> ous answer is: consume less cholesterol. Superficially this sounds
> like a good suggestion; actually it is a poor one. Most of our good
> foods contain substantial amounts of cholesterol, and if we try to
> eliminate cholesterol consumption we sacrifice good nutrition. In
> effect we would throw out the baby with the bath water. Anyone

who deliberately avoids cholesterol in his diet may be inadvertently courting heart disease.

As we shall see later, the evidence points to the conclusion that good nutrition, if it is really good, prevents cholesterol deposits from forming, even when our cholesterol consumption is moderately high. We must remember that cholesterol is made within our bodies, and that this homemade cholesterol can be deposited in the arteries of a person who consumes no cholesterol at all. Furthermore, the rate of synthesis of cholesterol in the body is inversely influenced by the available supply of cholesterol from outside (feedback mechanism). Not consuming cholesterol may in effect open the valve which accelerates the production of cholesterol within the body thereby increasing cholesterol synthesis.

Recently Random House published an important book exposing the cholesterol fairy tale: *Heart Failure. A Critical Inquiry into American Medicine and the Revolution in Heart Care* by Thomas J. Moore.

Elliot Corday, M.D., Clinical Professor of Medicine, UCLA School of Medicine, Los Angeles had this to say about the book:

> This exciting new book should help create a much needed debate on the cholesterol controversy and clarify the legal issues that are apt to follow. It is irresponsible to force the public into a costly cholesterol-reducing program without firm scientific evidence of its effectiveness.

It's significant that the book was put out by Random House, a publisher which not only has a reputation as a responsible house but brings out many books each year sponsored by the American Medical Association.

An article by Thomas J. Moore covering the same information was published in the September 1989 *Atlantic*, a highly responsible magazine that painstakingly vets its articles.

Edward R. Pinckney, M.D., a former editor of the *Journal of the American Medical Association*, and Russell L. Smith, Ph.D. have written a most important book on the subject of cholesterol entitled *Diet, Blood Cholesterol and Coronary Heart Disease: A Critical Review of the Literature* (published by Vector Enterprises, Inc., Santa Monica, Calif. 1989).

These two responsible scientists undertook the gargantuan task of reading, reviewing, picking apart and analyzing 1700 scientific articles about cholesterol that appeared in peer-reviewed medical journals. Their conclusions are so important they must be quoted:

> The National Heart, Lung and Blood Institute (NHLBI) and the American Heart Association (AHA) are involved in a massive campaign to convince all Americans that diet is a major cause of high blood cholesterol levels and coronary heart disease (CHD). This report is a comprehensive and critical review of nearly 1700 medical research articles and reports, including food consumption trend studies, dietary cholesterol and fat experiments and clinical trials. In addition, literature relating CHD with alcohol, exercise, aspirin and fish oils is also critically reviewed. Also, a detailed discussion of the effects and potential effects of cholesterol-lowering and cholesterol-lowering agents is presented.
>
> It is concluded that diet is, at best, only negligibly related to CHD, particularly for the vast majority of persons. Moreover, all the major epidemiological studies reveal an extremely weak relationship between blood cholesterol and CHD, often showing an increase in annual CHD rate of less than one percent across most or all of the blood cholesterol range. This fact alone indicates that diet cannot possibly have more than a very minor influence on CHD.
>
> A major reason why diet and blood cholesterol *appear* to be important determinants of CHD is because data are often presented in unorthodox ways, weak data are often interpreted as "powerful," and numerous reviews of the literature are invariably incomplete and strongly biased. In fact, the majority of relevant literature is either ignored or erroneously cited as supporting the diet-blood cholesterol-CHD relationship. While NHLBI and AHA frequently state that the evidence "overwhelmingly" supports the relationship, clearly the reverse is true. It does not seem possible that objective scientists without vested interests could ever interpret the literature as supportive.

Translation

Translating their front-parlor English, they're saying: The scientists who keep pumping up the cholesterol monster have been bought off.

When attempting to find a criminal, the French police have a saying: *Cherchez la femme*. Translation: *Look for the woman*.

When trying to find the force behind a popular push in the world of nutrition, I have a saying: *Cherchez l'argent* (*Look for the money*).

Once upon a time when our ancestors crawled out of their cave in the morning, they faced obvious and comparatively harmless foes like saber-toothed tigers, or a gang of warriors from the other side of the mountain coming to bang them in the head with a stone axe and carry off their women along with any valuables lying around the cave like cured skins and stone tools.

Such were our ancestors' rather obvious, old-fashioned enemies. Our ancestors expected them. They took precautions against them.

Today much more dangerous enemies stalk us. Like computer viruses, today's unnoticed enemies use advertising to dive into our minds and leave in place ideas that multiply and control us so that we smile happily as we voluntarily hand over that which belongs to us, our money and our lives.

For 2.2 million years (146,000 generations) our ancestors ate a diet of fresh meat along with its fat, plus a few vegetables and fruits. Thus evolution designed our body chemistry to deal with such a diet.

Man started eating new foods such as grains and milk products in important amounts only during the past 5,000 to 10,000 years (350 generations). Table sugar came along only 150 years (five generations) ago.

Evolution has not yet had time to completely alter our biochemistry to handle the new foods.

Conclusion

It's been fashionable to blame high serum cholesterol levels in part on eating animal fats. I have strong evidence, however, that the real problem comes from eating animal fats *plus* the new foods such as grains, milk products, and sugar. *The new foods seem to block the body's ability to handle animal fats.*

The American Heart Association speculates that the death rate from coronary attacks is going down because people are eating less fat.

Linus Pauling, a two-time Nobel Prize-winning scientist, and I both agree that the heart attack rate is falling because every year people are taking more vitamin C.

18

Meat Versus Wheat

The mass distrusts controversy. Reluctant to reconsider its convictions, superstitions, and prejudices, it rarely withdraws support for those who are guiding its destinies. Thus inertia becomes an incumbent's accomplice. So does human reluctance to admit error. Those who backed the top man insist, against all evidence, that they made the right choice.

— WILLIAM MANCHESTER

"Meat has impurities in it!" readers will complain.

Please, do you think I'm naive?

Today, everything we take into our bodies has impurities in it. New York has 200 chemicals in its drinking water. Some of them are radioactive.

Eighty-seven percent of nursing mothers have PCBs in their milk. Also, mother's milk is radioactive. The radiation is so high that it's not legal for a wet nurse to travel from one state to another to sell her milk. It doesn't meet federal milk standards!

Everything we eat is a compromise. Even with its impurities, however, most babies do best on mother's milk.

It's the same with meat. In spite of its impurities, many people do best on a diet with large amounts of fish, poultry or red meat.

If you think meat is impure, what about wheat? A wheat farmer who consulted me told me what happens to the wheat grown on her farm. They spray wheat with chemicals many times while in the field. Farmers spray it again with chemicals when it goes to the silo to keep away mice. They spray wheat with chemicals to prevent fungus growth. They spray chemicals such as Tetrafume yet again to keep out insects.

157

They mix last year's moldy wheat with this year's fresh wheat so the inspectors will miss the bad wheat.

The mold *Aspergillus* is often found in wheat, grains, nuts, grapes, peanut butter, bread, cheese, apple juice. This mold forms aflatoxins. Aflatoxins are among the most reliable causes of liver cancer.

Bakers add more chemicals when they make flour into bread. I read the chemicals listed on the wrapper of a loaf of bread: lactylate, monoglycerides, biglycerides, polyglycerate 60, polysorbatego, potassium bromide, artificial flavorings. The words "artificial flavorings" may mean dozens of chemicals. Artificial apple flavoring may contain 183 different chemicals!

And remember, there is no requirement to list *all* the chemicals used. Bread contains hundreds of other chemicals such as bleaches, dough strengtheners, firming agents, leavening agents . . . and on and on until bread appears to have every chemical known to man.

Pyrrolizidine alkaloids are found in many plants. These plants grow in wheat fields. Often farmers harvest the plants with the wheat and pyrrolizidines contaminate the wheat. Pyrrolizidines have killed people. Scientists have linked pyrrolizidines with liver cancer.

The phytic acid in seeds and grains (including wheat) binds calcium, magnesium, zinc and copper. It prevents the absorption of these important minerals.

Mellanby learned that the binding of calcium by phytic acid in wheat helps bring on rickets (bone deformities) in children. This is the same wheat found in cake, cookies, bread and breakfast cereals.

Eating grains (such as wheat) causes the body to lose calcium in bones and helps bring on osteoporosis (calcium-weak bones that easily break). This explains many hip fractures in older women.

Because phytic acid also binds magnesium, it prevents the body from absorbing magnesium. A low body level of magnesium can cause irregular heartbeat (and many other heart problems) and other difficulties such as poor appetite (anorexia), nausea, and periods of overactivity and lack of energy. Low magnesium levels tend to cause low body levels of calcium and potassium.

Other medical and psychological difficulties attributed to a magnesium deficiency include: convulsions in infants, personality changes, muscle spasm, restlessness, high suicide rate, anorexia nervosa and bulimia.

Drinking alcoholic beverages makes magnesium deficiencies worse.

The low zinc levels caused by the binding of zinc by phytic acid injures the body's immune system. This makes people more likely to get infections (including AIDS) and more susceptible to cancer.

Because phytic acid from grains lowers copper levels, it may cause some forms of anemia. Copper deficiency lowers T-cell antigens in rats. Low copper levels may contribute to some forms of arthritis, cancer, allergies and still more health problems.

Recently Memorial Sloan-Kettering Cancer Institute surprised the medical world by publishing research indicating that calcium added to the diet protects against cancer of the bowel. As mentioned, phytic acid in grains (including wheat and wheat products) cuts down on the absorption of calcium. Thus, eating wheat probably helps bring about bowel cancer.

Dohan and others from the University of Pennsylvania agree with me. They found that the gluten in wheat may cause schizophrenia— especially the paranoid type—in certain people.

We sell our wheat to the Russians, which makes them more paranoid. Then we spend billions to defend ourselves against them!

Vegetarians should build a shrine to Hitler, the world's most famous vegetarian. Hitler was a great wheat eater. For breakfast he had toast and chocolate.

Vegetarians frequently are deficient in vitamin B12 and develop brain damage from their B12 deficiency. If Hitler had eaten meat or had been given a few dollars' worth of vitamin B12 injections, World War II might have been avoided.

Bugs for Breakfast, Anyone?

There's no limit to the number of dead insect bodies flour may have in it. The number of dead insect wings, legs, heads and tails in a bowl of breakfast cereal or a loaf of bread is astronomical. Insects are highly allergenic.

The government allows two *rat* pellets per 1000 grams of wheat, about a quart. Rat pellets are many times larger than mouse droppings. These rat pellets are in the wheat used to make bread—even in your beloved whole wheat bread—breakfast cereals, spaghetti and cake.

In susceptible people, I have seen wheat—and its common contaminants—incompatibilities produce almost every disease you can name, including tension, paranoid schizophrenia, high blood pressure, depression, arthritis, asthma and many more.

I once thought that table sugar was the biggest nutritional problem in our modern world. Having studied and treated thousands of patients for diseases caused by their incompatibility with wheat, observations have led me to conclude that wheat is our biggest problem. Other grains follow close behind it. In a sense table sugar is also a grain. Most of it comes from sugar cane, which is a relative of corn, a grain.

People look upon breakfast as a special meal. Most people eat a breakfast cereal or a roll for breakfast. Both contain wheat. People who have eaten no wheat overnight are beginning to have withdrawal symptoms from not eating wheat. They're ready for their wheat fix first thing in the morning. They "just don't feel right" without it.

If you feel passionate about wheat, as most people do in the Western world, you are probably addicted to it, as most people are in the Western world.

People who use heroin feel passionate about heroin. Cocaine users feel passionate about cocaine. We need a government that will protect us against the wheat growers and pushers.

19

Meat, Fat and Cancer

> *Vitamin C may turn out to be the most important of all nutrients in the control of cancer, but others are also important.*
>
> —LINUS PAULING

You hear that diets high in animal fats *might* contribute to breast or bowel cancer. Such information is gathered by epidemiologists. Epidemiologists are scientists who study, among other things, the relationship between illness and factors which may produce illness. Unfortunately, epidemiologists often do not know enough about their subject. As a result, they often study and report on meaningless generalities.

Many people, to serve their own ends, seize on the pseudo-facts handed out by epidemiologists and present them as if they were hard facts.

Epidemiologists might study deaths in New York City and correlate the deaths with what people drank during the year prior to their death. A paper resulting from such a study might report:

1. In the city of New York, 151 people died during the week of June 23–29, 1990.

2. Of those who died, 149 of the people drank city water within 12 months of the time of their death.

Because you are acquainted with city water, you will read the above facts and say, "So what? That doesn't make sense."

The chances are, however, that you know little about *fats* and *meats* and *cancer*, so you would not see through "facts" about them so easily.

161

Interested parties seize upon pseudo-facts put out by epidemiologists and used the pseudo-facts for their own ends. The *Anti-Democratic Gazette* published in Beijing might read the "facts" about deaths in the city of New York and print a story that would say: "The democratic government in the city of New York killed 149 of its citizens last week by giving them city water to drink!"

Epidemiologists whose work I have read and with whom I have spoken do not know nearly enough about the subjects of meats, fats and cancer to collect meaningful data. They pay far too *little attention to details.* Here are some of the mistakes they make:

1. Epidemiologists dump all animal fats together: the fat on meat that has aged for two weeks in the butcher's refrigerator, unaged meats, meats with preservatives such as hot dogs and salami, darkly browned meat, smoked meats, ground meats (which oxidize quickly) and others.

2. Epidemiologists do not separate meats cooked with gas from meats cooked with electricity.

3. Epidemiologists do not measure the vitamin-mineral levels of the people they study.

4. Epidemiologists do not record the vitamin-mineral intake of their subjects.

5. Epidemiologists do not record all of the foods that their subjects eat, whether they are eating wheat (for example), which cuts down on the absorption of calcium and thus (according to a recent paper published from Sloan-Kettering Cancer Center) increases cancer of the colon.

Breakfast cereal hucksters gather the incorrect, pseudo-scientific data put out by epidemiologists, add the word "may" to avoid legal difficulties, and use the information to sell their products.

"Cutting down the fat in the diet *may* reduce your risk of cancer," the pseudo-nice man in the TV ad says.

He says the word "may" very softly so you, in effect, hear, "Cutting down the fat in the diet reduces your risk of cancer."

Thus false information is implanted in an entire society. Lies becomes truths.

As the *Congressional Record* stated in August, 1976, many researchers who come out against eating meat get their research and personal money from food manufacturers. Most of the manufacturers want to discourage meat eating. They want people to eat the high-profit foods they make: grain products such as breakfast cereals.

Even meat producers would rather sell you processed meats such as salami or hot dogs. It's easier to ship and handle processed meat because it has a longer shelf life. More important, the markup is higher than on fresh meat. The percentage profit is greater.

The Facts

Breast cancer is much more common in women who are overweight. Cancer of the bowel occurs more frequently in overweight people. The best way to lose weight is to eat fewer carbohydrates such as wheat and sugar. As this book illustrates, eating a diet high in animal fats usually results in weight loss.

Please forgive me if I repeat some of these critically important points. Years of clinical experience and many scientific facts made me decide that people can safely eat a high-meat, high-animal-fat diet if they take these precautions.

1. Eat meat that is fresh, unaged and unpreserved. Especially should people avoid smoked meat or meat with nitrites in it.

Aging oxidizes fat. Oxidized fat is a troublemaker. Not only does it destroy certain vitamins and make foods harder to utilize, but oxidized fats cause cancer in some people.

We have known for many years that smoked foods cause cancer. The stomach juices change the nitrites in nitrite-preserved meats into nitrosamines. Nitrosamines are powerful cancer producers.

2. The possible risk from meat and animal fat comes not from the fresh meat and fat itself, but from *oxidized* fat. Aging (exposure to the air) and browning or burning oxidizes fats.

For years I have made the clinical observation that most patients feel best on marbleized fresh meat, such as beef rib steak. One of the reasons is that oxygen does not reach the central marbleized fat.

Thicker cuts also have less fat exposed to the air.

Do not eat the fat around the outer (1/8 inch) edge of the meat.

The fat is especially suspect if you burn the fat.

Fat (in red meats, chickens, eggs, etc.) oxidizes even if you refrigerate it immediately after cooking.

When cooks keep vegetable cooking oils (fats) hot and use them over and over again, the fats are cancer-producing. This often happens in restaurants where they French-fry foods.

Boiling meat briefly gives the least oxidized fat. Boiling is also the fastest—faster even than microwave cooking—and the least expensive way to cook. Most people react better to the meat if they leave it pink in the center. Of course, you must cook pork well.

Some people can tolerate meat only if they boil it. *Browned and burned fats and meats are chemically different from the original fats and meats, just as rust is a different chemical from iron.*

Baking overheats the fat and is not an acceptable way to cook. The same is true of cooking in convection ovens. Microwave cooking is very tricky. Avoid it.

If broiled, meat should be only lightly browned. Scrape and/or cut away any browned or burned sections.

Pan-frying is the most suspect way to cook meat. Frying subjects the meat to a high temperature. If you eat pan-fried meat, fry it slowly so it's not burned. If burned or browned, scrape and cut away the browned and burned part.

Some people feel best on raw meat, steak tartare. Nureyev, the ballet star, is a good example. If you do eat raw meat, it's best to keep it frozen for three days, then thaw and eat it.

3. No one should cook meat with gas. Like automobile fumes, gas is a hydrocarbon. Gas gets into meat, especially into the fat. For more than a hundred years we have known that hydrocarbons cause cancer.

4. Much research shows that adequate vitamins A, C, carotene, choline, E, folic acid, zinc and selenium are especially protective against cancer.

Recently, researchers have added vitamin B6 to the list, after two current studies by the Louisiana State University Medical Center and the Massachusetts Institute of Technology. A 1985 study from Memorial Sloan-Kettering Cancer Institute showed that a generous intake of calcium also protects against bowel cancer.

Scientific papers continue to stress the importance of vitamins and minerals for the prevention of cancer. Epidemiologists who ignore this fact are living in Never-Never Land.

If you heed most food advertising, you too are living in Never-Never Land. Check your pocket: Someone may have a hand in it.

20

Meat Phobia

People are tyrannized by their culture.

—EDWARD T. HALL

Everybody "knows" that red meat is bad for you. How do they know? They just know. They "know" like the Cuban schoolchild "knows" that democracy is bad. Everybody says so.

People think I favor eating red meat. Not true. *I don't care what people eat as long as it's compatible with their individual chemistry.*

The other day a patient walked into my office, sat down and smiled.

"That cod liver oil you asked me to take is the best thing I ever tasted," he said.

Curious about his chemistry, I asked about his family background. Both of his parents came from a seacoast town in Norway. His family had always lived there. Probably they had been eating a fish diet for thousands of years. Many generations ago those who could not thrive on a fish diet either left or died. The ones who survived had chemistries that could thrive on fish. They passed that chemistry along to their children, and on down generation to generation.

I told myself that any patient who liked cod liver oil might do better on fish than on red meat.

I switched the patient back and forth between a high beef diet and

165

a high fish diet. He felt better on fish. He could eat beef only once a week. Eating pork and lamb gave him a headache and made him tired. He felt great on fish.

I don't care what people eat so long as it's right for their individual chemistry.

When You Challenge Conventional Wisdom

After Marconi announced that he could send messages through air, they thought he was mad. Today everyone accepts radio transmission.

I remember in the movie houses during the 1930s the news shorts showed scientists launching rockets. The rockets would lift a few hundred feet, fizzle out and fall to earth. Everyone would laugh. They stopped laughing when Hitler began firing rockets that landed on London.

Whenever something new comes along, the world regularly laughs at it and rejects it.

Many people do not thrive in our world. Such people crowd doctors' offices, swallow pills by the millions and fill hospital beds. Most of them remain ill. They only get treatment for their symptoms.

For example, if a man has high blood pressure, he gets pills that reduce his pressure. To keep his pressure down, he must continue taking the pills. His doctor treats the symptom; he does not cure him.

I find that food incompatibilities and an inadequate supply of vitamins, minerals and unsaturated fats cause almost all high blood pressure. An incompatibility with sugar and/or wheat is by far the most common cause of high blood pressure. Among patients who follow my directions, I can't remember failing to cure a single patient with high blood pressure.

How do I know? I have tried thousands of patients on different combinations of foods. These were patients suffering from common medical ailments such as asthma, arthritis, backache, Crohn disease, lupus, migraine headaches, peptic ulcers, thalassemia and many others. Most of these patients made the rounds of other doctors' offices before visiting me. Many had also been to famous private clinics without finding relief.

I am sorry that so many people do well on red meats. Many readers will not believe me. My observations will offend other people.

I suspect when Harvey discovered that blood circulated he knew other physicians would laugh at him. Blood, however, did circulate. He had no choice but to report his findings.

Why do many patients feel better on meat? I'm not sure, but I suspect part of the answer is that red meat, especially beef, is the closest to the ancestral food mankind has eaten for 2.2 million years. It's the food for which evolution designed our chemistry.

The medical profession loses sight of an important fact. Evolution is not something that happened a long time ago to funny-looking hairy people. Evolution still goes on.

Evolution has given us people with widely varying body chemistries. Those of us (like me) who have primitive chemistries can only handle primitive foods like a fish-fowl-meat-vegetable-fruit diet.

We become ill (and/or fat) if we eat a modern diet of grains, sugar and milk.

Some people in our modern world with modern chemistries can thrive (and maintain a normal weight) on pizza, ice cream and hot dogs. So be it. Then let them eat the modern goodies. I only wish I could.

One of the problems with the medical profession: It fails to distinguish between people with modern chemistries and people with primitive chemistries.

I've heard all the arguments about red meat. We've covered some of the objections in the three previous chapters. Let's talk more about the problem.

Reasons Why People Reject Red Meat

Historical

1. Red meat first met with disfavor in Europe during the Middle Ages (500 A.D. to 1500 A.D.) when most of the people living in towns and cities were too poor to afford meat. *People enjoy eating what they learn to eat as children.* Chinese children like bird's nest soup. French children enjoy snails. People came to prefer wheat products and to reject meat.

2. The early settlers in this country ate food shipped in from England, including salt pork and beef. They learned that eating salt meat led to scurvy, a deadly disease that comes from a lack of vitamin C. They blamed the meat. In part, they were correct. Fresh red meat protects people from scurvy, but salted meat does not.

The Indians taught the Hudson Bay Company trappers to eat pemmican, a mixture of dried buffalo or caribou meat and melted fat. This unsalted, uncooked form of red meat prevented scurvy. It even cured scurvy.

By the time the early settlers learned the difference between eating fresh and salted meat, it was too late. Already they had decided that meat was "bad for you." The idea became a part of society's conventional wisdom.

3. During the early days of this country, savage Indians and rough frontiersmen killed buffalo and lived off buffalo meat. The more refined town and city people, however, dined off freshly baked bread, casseroles, sweets and other "civilized" foods.

Women thought it more elegant to cook and serve foods other than red meat. They didn't want their husbands to eat like roughnecks. They didn't want their children to eat meat and grow up like savages and uncouth frontiersmen.

Women came to reject red meats and to embrace "high class" foods. The children and the men ate what the women prepared.

4. Many women enjoy cooking: making blueberry pancakes, baking bread and pies, decorating cakes. Then, as now, women enjoyed making food more attractive and more appetizing. Red meat does not easily lend itself to such improvements.

Social

1. Old wives' tales say that red meat will give you arthritis, will cause hardening of the arteries and help bring on heart attacks and strokes. They say red meat will give you cancer of the breasts and colon, bring on high blood pressure, put a strain on the kidneys. In mysterious, unknown ways it will wreck havoc with your system.

Strange as it may sound, scientists, including nutritionists and physicians, also believe those old wives' tales.

The old wives' tales simply are not true. Professors gave Vilhjalmut Stefansson those same arguments when he and a friend entered Bellevue

Hospital here in New York to put themselves on an all-meat diet for a year.

The chief reason scientists speak out against red meat is that they do not understand addiction to wheat. They fail to correctly diagnose withdrawal symptoms that appear when people stop eating wheat and sugar.

2. Red meats require cooking. The modern woman doesn't spend as much time cooking as did her mother and her grandmother.

Today's woman often has a nine-to-five job plus her housework. She is badly overworked and has only the time and energy to serve prepared or semi-prepared foods.

3. Some "liberated" women feel put upon if they spend any time in the kitchen.

Psychological

1. Many people in this country feel that killing animals and eating meat is morally wrong.

Crowded together in cities, living shoulder-to-shoulder with strangers, mankind inhibits his killer instincts. Subconsciously, he associates killing animals with killing his fellow man. Thus he rejects meats.

2. Since the Mayflower days, we have held the puritan's view that if a thing is pleasurable it's sinful. People in this country have always enjoyed eating juicy broiled steaks. Therefore, eating steaks must be bad!

3. Mankind is a clever animal who has learned to fly from New York to Paris in three hours. He can send colored pictures through the air. He has blasted astronauts to the moon. Mistakenly, mankind feels that because he understands the laws of nature, he can ignore them. Man has come to see himself as a god who is above the laws of nature. He believes that he is all mind and spirit. He forgets that, like a dog or horse, he too has a body chemistry. In his arrogance, man has come to believe that the food he eats is of little importance.

If you owned a million-dollar racehorse, would you try to take him off his ancestral diet of grain? Would you feed him oat-flavored hot dogs and steaks? On such a diet would he win any races?

You say you wouldn't feed your valuable horse that way?

Then why do you feed your even more valuable children a diet that leaves their brains so scrambled they cannot concentrate on schoolwork, a diet that leaves them feeling so miserable that in ever greater numbers they commit suicide?

The teenage suicide rate has doubled since 1968, largely because mothers demonstrate their love by keeping the refrigerators stocked with sugary soda drinks and feed them cereals for breakfast and spaghetti for dinner. Their grandparents bring them candy and ice cream. Why do we insist upon rotting the brains of a whole generation of children, turning them into scholastic failures, delinquents, dropouts and welfare recipients? Why do we drive more and more of them to suicide by feeding them ever more processed foods? I'll tell you why: Many people are getting rich at their expense.

We look askance at African tribes when they cut faces and rub dyes into the wounds and when they circumcise women. That's child's play compared to what we do to our children.

In our society, it's perfectly all right to maim and kill—so long as we do it in a socially acceptable way.

Political

1. Our government helps spread the falsehood that we need a varied diet. Washington tells us to eat little red meat.

Let's pretend that you work in the Department of Agriculture and your supervisor asks you to write a pamphlet telling people how to choose a correct diet. How would you go about it?

First, you might ask yourself how you could please your supervisor and put yourself in line for a promotion. To avoid criticism, you would try not to challenge conventional wisdom. You would not go against what "everybody knows to be true."

To stay on the safe side, you would consult a professor of nutrition at one of the leading universities. Never mind that the professor knows much about the food chemistry of laboratory mice, but has little practical, direct information about human nutrition. Of course, the professor knows nothing about food incompatibilities and wheat addiction. He doesn't want to know. He too is addicted to wheat.

As long as you quote a Harvard professor, no one can blame you if the information is wrong. You're clean. You'll get your promotion.

As a government worker putting together a booklet on nutrition, you would not mention that milk makes 70 percent of African-Americans and Orientals (and at least 30 percent of Caucasians) ill. If you said that, the milk lobby would howl for your scalp.

You wouldn't tell people to eat red meat. That would offend the cereal manufacturers and the sugar lobby.

In any case, the government cannot admit that a high-animal-fat, high-animal-protein diet is healthful. For one thing, there's not enough meat and animal fat to feed everyone.

Medical

1. Cholesterol is the undesirable type of fat in the bloodstream. Many studies suggest that people with high cholesterol levels die younger. They have more strokes and heart attacks. The people studied were eating the "average American diet," diets that included table sugar, milk products and grains.

The medical profession has decided that red meat—high in animal fat—raises the serum cholesterol and therefore is undesirable.

The profession is wrong.

As I have detailed in Chapter 17, it is not the high animal fat diet that makes the serum cholesterol go up. It's the lack of proper vitamins, minerals, and other nutritional supplements. It's the lack of physical activity. It's eating grains, sugar, and milk products along with the fat that makes the cholesterol climb when eating animal fat.

I sent a paper based on my research to the editor of the *Journal of the American Medical Association.* Also, I mailed a copy to the editor of a journal published by the American Heart Association. Because my findings are at odds with their conventional wisdom, each rejected it. They said they already had too many papers awaiting publication.

It pleased me when the *International Journal for Vitamin and Nutrition Research* in Switzerland published the paper. The publication resulted in worldwide interest. Later this year a longer version will appear in the *Southern Medical Journal.*

2. I want to repeat: Most professors of nutrition in this country do not know much about *human* nutrition. They spend their lives doing research on white mice or rabbits. Since both the mouse and the rabbit are largely vegetarians, the conclusions reached are not valid for humans.

Unfortunately, researchers conduct their experiments on animals that drink chlorinated and fluoridated water. They confine the animals to small cages so they have very little exercise. They give them no full-spectrum light. These abnormal conditions distort the animals' normal biochemistry. The findings are not even valid for mice and rabbits!

3. Don't bother to ask the average physician about nutrition. He knows less than his receptionist about it. The doctor, however, will put a wise-in-the-ways-of-health-matters expression on his face. He will then give the standard answer used by those who know nothing about the subject, "Just eat the average American diet. . . ."

That's good advice if you want average American health: obesity, high blood pressure, premature senility, heart disease and cancer.

4. A doctor consulted me because of pain in his legs. He talked about his leg muscles' need for more oxygen.

It confused the doctor when I asked, "What about your muscles' need for calcium, magnesium and vitamins?"

His medical training has imprisoned his mind. They taught him about a muscle's need for oxygen but said little about a muscle's need for vitamins and minerals.

Economic

1. The public has a false notion about medical researchers. They see these scientists as dedicated intellectuals, men and women who wear glasses because they've ruined their eyes reading weighty books. They are thin and have dark circles under their eyes. Night and day they slave in their laboratories to uncover nature's secrets.

A few scientists are like that. Such scientists live mostly in Mel Brooks' movies.

Recently I visited one of the world's great research centers. A glance at the bulletin board next to the main bank of elevators tells a great deal about scientists. The board was heavy with pinned-up cards that read:

"Wanted—weekend rides to ski area. Will share expenses."

"Baby-sitter desperately needed—mostly for Friday nights."

"For sale: almost new bassinet and baby carriage."

"Tennis anyone at 2 p.m. several afternoons a week?"

As you see, for the most part scientists are like other people. They like to recreate. At night when the lights go off, they have sex. They need more money.

Also, they have a need to move ahead in life. This means they must do research that will allow them to get papers published. Published papers help them step up from assistant professor to associate professor. They will earn more money and have more power. To do the research and write the papers, they must compete with each other for research money.

As in all competitive worlds, the world of nutritional research is less than honorable. Recently one of my patients—a medical student—spent the summer working in the laboratory of one of New York's leading medical schools. He observed the researchers reworking their data until they got them to come out in a way that would help them get more research funds. The primary purpose of their research was not to gather more knowledge, but to land more funds.

The biggest problem, however, is that the scientists themselves are usually addicted to wheat and sugar. If a scientist addicted to heroin does research on heroin, you can bet that he'll find good things to say about the drug. He's not going to advocate banning it from the face of the earth!

Several years ago when I appeared on a TV program, I got into an argument with an overweight nutritionist. He could not talk about food without getting red-in-the-face passionate. He was arguing about foods that had addicted him. From his passionate tone, you would think I was talking about his sex life or his mother's virtue.

How could such an addicted man do objective research about food?

2. The *Congressional Record* pointed out that Frederick Stare, professor of nutrition at Harvard, has accepted research funds from various food manufacturers. The *Congressional Record* said that food processing companies pay him a large personal salary for consulting with their boards of directors.

Dr. Stare was at that time on the board of directors of food companies that put sugar in their canned beans. Which is Dr. Stare going to advocate, red meat or his company's sugar-laced canned beans? How do you think he will advise congressional committees seeking his advice?

3. As pointed out earlier, even the meat industry would rather process meat into hot dogs or salami. That way they have fewer storage problems and make more profit per pound.

4. Companies make more money by selling easily packaged products like grains and sugar. That's why we see their expensive ads on prime-time TV.

Advertising companies have learned to keep repeating their message. People will believe anything if you tell it often enough. Hitler learned that repetition could turn a lie into the truth, into conventional wisdom.

Through television commercials, admen paid by the grain industry constantly whisper to us: Breakfast cereals are fun. Breakfast cereals give you vitamins. If you love your husband and children, you will feed them breakfast cereals.

George Orwell's 1984 has arrived. Bad is Good!

Physiological

1. Modern diets leave so many women tired and depressed that they cannot find the energy needed to cook.

2 In this country 30 million women are taking tranquilizers or antidepressants. (Sorry, I don't have the figures on men.) Often they simply do not feel up to cooking.

3. During prehistoric times, men were the hunters. They killed the animals and carried home the meat. Men were the combatants, the killers. Perhaps that explains why today's men like to watch football and boxing.

Women were the non-killers. They helped gather foods such as berries, roots, and nuts. In more recent times, they tended the fires and cooked the food. They loved their man and their children and thus assured the future of the race. Perhaps that's why women reject football and boxing and enjoy watching love stories.

Women are taking an ever stronger role in our present society, probably because their chemistry is tougher than men's. Females can better survive our present environment of chemical pollutants. They probably do better than men on our diet of hot dogs, sugar-laced cola drinks and cream-and-preservative-filled cupcakes.

With the domination of our society by females comes her more passive philosophy. Love, rather than killing for food, has always been woman's specialty. Killing—even the killing of barnyard animals—and the eating of red meat doesn't fit a philosophy based on love.

4. A dog or a cat or a horse—and almost all other animals except the guinea pig, fruit-eating bats, the higher apes and man—can make their own vitamin C.

At some very distant time the common ancestor of the higher apes and man suffered a mutation that lost his ability to make his own vitamin C. That was long before man became a meat eater 2.2 million years ago. Our ancestor ate so much fruit (and thus had vitamin C) that he had no need for the body to make its own. We could use our chemical machinery for more important tasks.

I speculate that at the same time our ancestor lost the ability to manufacture his own vitamin C, he developed an inborn taste for sweets.

At that time our ancestor couldn't stroll to the corner deli and buy a Baby Ruth bar. Sweets meant fruit. Evolution gave our ancestor a taste for sweets (fruits) so we would eat a steady supply of vitamin C-bearing fruits.

Today, manufacturers of sugar-rich foods and drinks have taken advantage of us. Instead of supplying us with fruit and vitamin C, they give us sugar-sprinkled breakfast cereals and sugar-laden drinks and cakes.

Unfortunately, these are the very foods that assure the medical profession an unending supply of patients.

5. *This is the most important point of all*: As discussed in Chapter Eight (that deals with food incompatibilities), grain and sugar addicts comprise a high percentage of the population. Once they hook us, the manufacturers have steady customers.

An addiction to grains or sugar is similar to an addiction to tobacco or heroin. Once we're hooked, we suffer withdrawal symptoms if we stop them. Withdrawal symptoms are unpleasant. They can range all the way from tiredness to headache, to muscle pains, to nausea, vomiting and diarrhea, to suicidally deep depressions.

To avoid these withdrawal symptoms, we continue to eat the grains and sugar. The force of addiction is stronger than the desire for a slender figure. It's stronger than honor, often stronger than life itself.

Conclusions

Man has a great need to explain why he does things. He thinks of reasons why he leaves home, why he marries, why he follows his occupation, why he eats certain foods and avoids others.

Primitive man explained the world in terms of the forest gods.

"Modern" Western man likes to give "scientific" reasons for his acts. If we do not have a scientific explanation, we invent one, often in the laboratory of a famous university. Our explanations—and those of scientists—eventually become a part of our culture's conventional wisdom.

People who reject red meat have too little knowledge about anthropology, about human nutrition, about human biochemistry.

People are truly tyrannized by their culture.

Red meat may be all wrong for you. It may be just the thing for you. Test yourself as directed in Chapter Eight and settle the question.

21

Constipation

A collision at sea spoils your whole day.
—CAPTAIN HAZELWOOD

Like obesity, tooth decay, high blood pressure and insomnia, constipation is a disease of civilization. I call such disorders *the Newbold Syndrome*.

Soft, tasty modern foods made with sugar and grains account for most constipation. Too few unsaturated fats in the diet and lack of exercise magnify the problem. Often those who are chronically constipated developed cancer of the colon.

Anyone with persistent constipation should have a gastroenterologist pass a colonoscope to view the large bowel and a barium enema X-ray.

Bran Isn't the Answer

In health food stores, I see shelves heavy with books telling about the glory of a high fiber diet. On TV, ads praise Brand X cereal because it's high in fiber.

True, bran helps the problem, but bran also creates new problems. Bran is not the way to go. Hardly a week passes without my seeing a patient who's been ill since starting to use bran. The problem is that

177

bran has wheat particles in it. Wheat is the single biggest problem food in the modern diet. It's the single largest cause of diseases such as tooth decay, arthritis, headaches, high blood pressure, lupus, schizophrenia— and dozens of others.

Bran interferes with the absorption of calcium, magnesium and other minerals. Thus it contributes to osteoporosis, cancer of the colon and certain types of heart disease.

Most so-called nutritionists find a bandwagon and jump on it. Next come the big-money cereal people. The best way to make money is to tell people easy ways to do difficult things—and to confirm their false beliefs.

It's amusing that the books on the shelf next to the "fiber" books talk about the glories of drinking "health-giving" juices. TV ads agree. Have you ever stopped to think that fruit and vegetable juices have no fiber? If fiber's so great, why not eat the whole fruit rather than drink fiber-free juices? Obviously, people have not thought through the problem.

Prevent Constipation

Raw fruits and raw vegetables, fats, magnesium, vitamin C, water and walking help prevent constipation in my patients. The most important way to prevent constipation, however, is to eat only foods that are compatible with your biochemistry.

As mentioned before, you should follow no diet advice without your physician's approval. Also, he or she should approve all vitamins, minerals and unsaturated oils you take.

You have already learned that I like my patients to eat only raw fruits and vegetables. These make a good source of fiber. Because of pesticides and other chemicals, however, people should eat them in limited amounts. Also, fruits and vegetables are often incompatible with people's biochemistries, especially if eaten in large amounts.

I ask my patients to have no more than half a cup of fresh, raw vegetable three times a day. They need to limit fresh raw fruit to one cup three times a day. Many people must cut out all fruit until they reach their ideal weight. *Many people with weight problems can never eat any fruits and do not tolerate root vegetables such as carrots.*

Fats

In one respect, fats act like fiber. Like fiber, fats also speed up the bowel transit time and reduce constipation. Most people reading this book will be eating fatty fish, the fatty skin on chicken and some of the fat on red meats. The fat will help prevent constipation.

In addition, they will have unsaturated fats like cod liver oil, safflower oil and linseed oil. If not incompatible with their biochemistries, my patients may have olive oil. These oils do much to help prevent problems with constipation.

Vitamin C and Magnesium

Except for a rare patient who is allergic to vitamin C and magnesium, I ask my patients to take them. I feel that both of these are more effective in the powder form.

I suggest that most of my patients take vitamin C powder. They do better on the fine type that's like flour, *not the coarse vitamin C that's like sugar.*

Most patients start with half a teaspoon of fine vitamin C powder in a glass of room-temperature water three times a day. If patients are still constipated, I may have them increase it to one teaspoon four times a day.

In addition, I ask them to take dolomite powder (calcium and magnesium), half a teaspoon three times daily. They may mix the dolomite powder with the vitamin C powder. If still constipated, I may have patients increase it to one teaspoon four times a day.

If you want to take powders with you when eating away from home, tear off squares of aluminum wrap. Place one dose of the vitamin C powder and one dose of the dolomite powder on the dull side of the foil. Twist the ends of the foil together and put it in your pocket. When ready to take it, simply tear the foil and shake it into a glass of water.

Many patients do better if they take magnesium oxide at bedtime, one or two 250 mg tablets of magnesium oxide. If this causes loose stools, stop taking it. Most patients sleep better if they take magnesium at bedtime. A rare patient feels hung over from it the next morning.

To regulate the bowels, switch back and forth between doses and combination of doses of vitamin C and dolomite. (Check your dolomite to be sure it does not have excessive amounts of heavy metals.)

Temporary Aids

When the patient begins his diet and supplements, he may need temporary help to relieve constipation. The insertion of a glycerine suppository is the easiest and least expensive first step. Often it's not enough to help the problem. Still, it's safe and deserves a try.

You don't need a prescription to go to the drugstore and buy an adult- (or child-) size glycerine suppository. Twenty minutes before you're ready for a bowel movement, hold a suppository under warm water for a moment to soften the surface. Squat and insert it all the way into the rectum.

If you have no bowel movement within an hour, you require stronger measures.

Enemas are more bothersome than suppositories. But like suppositories, they are not likely to cause trouble. *Do not use the prepared enemas that drugstores sell.* Do not use harsh liquids such as coffee or soapsuds. The point is to solve the problem without bringing on new problems. Use bottled spring water. Add exactly one measuring teaspoon of ordinary table salt to each quart. Warm the water.

Use a gravity-type enema bag, the type you hang on a hook. Pour the water into the bag. Hang the enema bag about three feet above your hips. Apply lubricating jelly to the tip of the nozzle at the end of the hose. Get in the tub on your knees and elbows. Insert the nozzle into your rectum. Unsnap the key that pinches the tube. If you can retain it, allow the entire quart of water to enter your colon. Then transfer to the toilet and do your thing.

If you have no results, repeat the enema once or twice. If you still get no results, either constipation is not your problem or you have a fecal impaction which may require medical treatment.

If you are allergic to something in your environment or to something you eat or drink, it can give you either diarrhea or constipation.

Frequent loose stools or chronic abdominal discomfort are almost always caused by incompatibilities. It's especially important that you consult your physician about such problems, however, to rule out other causes, such as cancer. Take care of your incompatibilities and that will solve the problem.

Every day drink at least a quart and a half of bottled spring water or water that you distill yourself. Do not use store-bought distilled water. Experience has taught me that patients usually do poorly on it.

22

If You Can't Walk, Crawl!

Why did they make our legs so long and our brains so short?

—H. L. Newbold

I was on my walk the other day when I happened across a 50-year-old, overweight woman who had tried to camouflage the misery showing in her face by applying pounds of white powder, red lipstick and purple eye shadow. She hobbled out of an apartment building. Her puffy skin was pale and unhealthy. She walked slowly and bent over, as if depressed and tired. Although I passed within three feet of her, she didn't notice me. She dwelled in her private land of misery and paid little attention to the world around her. As if she could hardly maneuver her legs, she struggled into a taxi the doorman had waiting for her.

GERTRUDE SETZER

As the taxi moved into traffic, I remembered her name: Gertrude Setzer. Gertrude had originally consulted me because of crippling pain in her right knee. She had been my patient for about a year when she stopped coming to visit me. Because she had made brilliant progress, I assumed she discontinued her visits because she was free of symptoms.

When I returned to the office, I looked up her chart.

Nearly bedridden from pain and swelling in her left knee, Gertrude had first consulted me two years previously. My diagnosis and the diagnosis of an orthopedist who had previously treated her was osteoarthritis (also called hypertrophic arthritis) of the right knee.

I made the following additional diagnoses of obesity, multiple food incompatibilities, marital discord and chronic depression.

What I Discovered

1. Gertrude walked and engaged in other physical activities as little as possible.
2. She had more pain in her knee whenever she ate anything that contained wheat.
3. Milk and milk products made her tired and depressed.
4. She was addicted to sugar, which gave her a *Type-B* weight problem. Also, sugar caused insomnia and recurrent night leg cramps.

Gertrude was a typical example of the Newbold Syndrome. She suffered from a group of degenerative diseases brought about by the civilization in which she lived.

Had she lived a mere 100,000 years ago she could not have spent her days in a recliner while munching bonbons and watching TV. Instead she would have lived in a group of perhaps 30 people. The men would leave the cave to hunt for meat. The women would walk to search for things to eat, young shoots, berries, and tubers. When the troop moved to find a better supply of animals to hunt and a less picked-over territory, the women carried their youngest child and the household goods and trudged along.

(Dear Reader, you only think you have a better life. The woman living 100,000 years ago enjoyed better health, was happier, had more and better sex and didn't have any Joneses to keep up with.)

Back in the days when everyone walked many hours a day and ate a fish-fowl-meat-limited vegetable, limited fruit diet, few people developed osteoarthritis.

Four factors caused Gertrude's osteoarthritis:

1. Lack of walking.
2. Eating wheat, sugar, and milk products, modern foods that were incompatible with her particular body chemistry.
3. Insufficient calcium and magnesium in her diet.
4. Lack of sufficient vitamins C and D.

I asked her to get out of her apartment and walk every day. She was to start with five minutes and increase the time by five minutes every week until she reached and hour and five minutes.

I put her on calcium, magnesium, vitamins C and D, along with other nutritional supplements.

By having her eat one food at a time in a controlled way, I learned that eating wheat inflamed her knee. Wheat was the most important cause of her arthritis. I also identified the foods to which she was addicted and which made her overweight, and removed them from her diet.

She cooperated and followed the diet I worked out for her. She lost all of the pain and swelling in her knee. Her depression melted away. Her energy increased. Her excess weight vanished along with her insomnia and the night pains in her legs.

Gertrude even enjoyed some return of marital harmony.

What Had Happened?

On the evening after seeing Gertrude on the street, I telephoned and told her that I often thought about her and wondered how she was getting along.

In icy tones, Gertrude informed me that she had a surgical replacement of her right knee. The news surprised me.

"What happened?" I asked. "The last time I saw you, you were doing very well."

"The pain came back."

"What happened—did you go off your diet and stop walking?"

"I'm sorry, but I don't want to talk about it."

"I always like to learn. If I did something wrong, I want to know."

"Doctor Newbold, I really don't care to talk about it. Thank you for calling. I must hang up now. Take care."

The next day I telephoned her husband at work.

"I suppose it's my fault," he told me. "Gertrude went off her diet and stopped walking when she happened to learn that I have a girlfriend."

"Why didn't she come back to see me?"

"I think she wanted to be sick to make me feel guilty. She had surgery. Thirty thousand dollars, would you believe it? And she's practically a cripple."

Textbooks say that Gertrude's type of "old age" arthritis is caused by wear and tear on the joint surfaces.

The other day I watched a TV program designed to bring doctors up to date on the latest treatments for osteoarthritis. (I sometimes watch such programs for laughs—but they usually leave me wanting to weep.)

The program showed physicians examining and treating patients suffering from osteoarthritis. Every one of the patients was overweight. Each had the passive, unhealthy appearance that people get when they sit and eat goodies and watch TV. In my view, the chief causes of painful osteoarthritis are lack of walking and eating modern foods.

A mechanical knee might leave Gertrude free of knee pain, but she'll never be able to walk an hour and five minutes a day as she should. She will only be able to hobble about. As a result, she will never be well. Next, she'll develop painful osteoarthritis in her neck, or back, or hips.

Lack of walking will contribute to other medical difficulties. For example, a return to a sedentary life had contributed to the return of her obesity. The obesity will make her more likely to develop breast cancer, cancer of the colon, and high blood pressure. It will hasten her death. Tragically, she's so depressed, she doesn't much care.

Gertrude and her surgeon have offended you. Because of her needless surgery (most surgery is needless) and because of similar surgery in tens of thousands of people, both your taxes and your health insurance rates go up.

More About Walking

In Europe people understand the importance of walking better than in the States. Swiss children living within two miles of school must walk. The authorities even forbid them to ride bicycles to school.

Most people sit at a desk to earn a living. They hop into their car and stop at a drive-in or at a grocery store for something to eat. Civilization has made food-gathering easy. As usual, when mankind solves one problem he creates a new one. Physical inactivity is one of the new problems. Lack of activity, especially lack of walking, increases both incompatibilities and weight problems.

As life evolved, it came to depend upon things around it such as warmth, sunlight, water, oxygen, proteins, fats, vitamins and minerals. Especially did our bodies come to depend upon walking.

Why Our Legs Are Long

The drought that struck the world during the late Miocene epoch (which extended from 23 million years ago until about five million years ago) shrank the rain forests that once extended all the way to what is modern day London. The drought became so severe that the Mediterranean Sea dried up.

When the fruit-bearing trees began disappearing, the easy life of our distant ancestors ended. They began walking over the grasslands to hunt and search for food. Walking saved them from starvation.

By four million years ago, our ancestors stood upright and walked on two feet. This freed their arms for more important tasks such as gathering food and carrying it back to the young.

For millions of years our ancestors had to walk long distances to find food. They had to burn calories to find more calories. They tried to do things the easy way. Conserving energy became second nature.

The human nature that we inherited from them still tells us to work no more than we must. Our nature tells us not to exercise, not to work. It says relax, lounge around with a drink in hand and watch TV.

Nowadays, instead of following our natural inclination to find ways to conserve energy, we must go against our nature. We must push ourselves to burn energy. We must find large and small ways to get more activity.

Instead of using the remote TV control, we need to walk over and change the station. We need to buy only a few groceries so we'll need to go shopping again. We should welcome yard work and housework. It's necessary for our health. I suspect women live longer than men in part because they commonly do more of the shopping and housework.

Not long ago a woman who lives on Park Avenue visited my office.

Her hair and face looked as if Charles of the Ritz had perfected them
less than an hour before. She wore diamonds and a mink coat (protected
by her bodyguard-chauffeur).

"Any other suggestions?" she asked as she stood up to leave.

"Only one," I said. "Every morning when your maid arrives, take
her upstairs and prop her up in bed. Then turn on the TV and bring
her a beer. While she's resting and enjoying TV, *you* dust and vacuum
the apartment and scrub the kitchen floor."

"You can't be serious!"

"That's my way of saying that to lose weight you must find ways
to increase your activity. I'll give you a diet and vitamins and minerals.
They'll help. You must find ways to increase your activity."

The patient opted for walking plus exercise classes.

Walking Creates Electrical Currents

Recent research from MIT, the University of Illinois, and the Institute of Physical and Chemical Research helps us understand the importance of walking.

Impact activity like walking jars the body. Walking causes a slight
bending of the minerals in living tissues. The bending of the minerals makes
streaming electrical and piezoelectrical currents in organs throughout
the body. Because of the jarring, walking brings about much more
electrical activity than other exercises. Walking is much superior to
swimming or to weight lifting. It's even better than the expensive exercise programs pushed by bulimic movie stars with pseudo-great
personalities!

Our bones and muscles and ligaments—to say nothing of our
brains and other organs—have come to depend upon walking to stay
healthy.

For more than half a century we've known that diabetics handle
foods better and need less insulin if they exercise. Exercise helps nor-
malize their chemistry.

The purpose of exercise is not primarily to burn calories. We must
walk forever to burn the calories in one slice of cake. Walking makes
people less allergic, and helps the body chemistry settle down and work
properly.

Walking vs. Running

Running is in fashion at the moment. In my view, walking is a much better form of exercise.

Anthropology Looks at Running

We can understand ourselves and find better health only if we keep looking back at our anthropological beginnings.

For four million years our ancestors have walked on two legs. In groups of 30 they wandered from place to place searching for something to eat. They ran only if forced to avoid danger, or during a last-minute charge to kill an animal they had stalked.

Evolution designed deer and elk and antelopes for running. Running is their best defense. An antelope can outrun a lion.

- ◆ Evolution designed us for walking. Man can't run well enough to depend upon it to avoid enemies. We can't outdistance even poor runners such as lions.
- ◆ Running puts excessive stress on joints and ligaments.
- ◆ Running strains the chemistry of the heart muscle. That's why you so often read about runners dropping dead.
- ◆ Chemical changes caused by running are so great they often make women stop menstruating.

Some people feel tense and emotionally upset after running. It's caused by a buildup of lactic acid in the body. Injecting lactic acid intravenously will throw these people into the same feeling of near panic. You can avoid the buildup of lactic acid by taking vitamin B1 (thiamine) 100 mg.

The same people who feel miserable after running usually feel great after walking.

Medical theory says that faulty plumbing causes heart attacks. When arteries close, they stop carrying food and oxygen to the heart muscle. As a result, a section of the heart muscle dies.

Running stresses the heart muscle, which makes extra blood vessels develop. If a runner has a heart attack, supposedly the extra arteries will be enough to feed the heart muscle. He's more likely to live.

That's theory, not fact.

Autopsies often show badly clogged heart arteries, yet the patient had no symptoms or evidence of heart damage.

I have reasons to believe that heart attacks usually don't come from plumbing problems. Most often, heart attacks happen because the chemistry of the heart muscle breaks down. The chemical problem causes the muscle to cramp, much as we may have a leg cramp. After the heart muscle cramps, the artery leading to the cramped section of ,the heart muscle goes into spasm and blocks up.

My Clinical Observations

I've had patients who feel angina pain (heart pain) only after eating a food—like ice cream—which is incompatible with their biochemistry.

The heart muscle is often injured by incompatible foods and environmental substances, though most cardiologists in this country are not aware of it. Recently I told a patient that an incompatibility caused his attacks of fast heart beating. He didn't believe me. Several cardiologists in Boston and New York had examined him and said nothing about incompatibilities.

Without mentioning my diagnosis, the patient consulted Professor Ottilio Master, Chief, Cardiovascular Unit, Royal Post Graduate Medical School, Hammersmith Hospital, London. After a week of examinations and tests, Dr. Master told the patient he was suffering from food incompatibilities.

The late Dr. Arthur F. Coca, one of the world's most distinguished allergists, Professor of Medicine at Columbia University, pointed out in his book *The Pulse Test* that the heart is a frequent target of food incompatibility reactions. Dr. Coca built a system for testing foods based on the speeding up of the heartbeat by eating incompatible foods.

After leaving off the foods that cause reactions, many patients report fast beating of their hearts when cheating on their diets.

I suspect food reactions often strike the heart muscle, cause pain and may bring on a "coronary."

Albert Owens would become depressed if he ate corn, wheat, sugar and many other common foods. Finally we worked out a diet which allowed him to function well. As time passed, he became more and more liberal with his diet. Finally, he had a coronary. After he recovered from the acute episode, he discovered that straying from his proper diet gave him chest pain.

Chemical problems other than incompatibilities can give heart pain. A few years ago I saw a patient who was having frequent severe attacks of angina. Her cardiologist recommended bypass surgery. As a last resort before surgery, she made an appointment with me.

I gave her an injection of vitamin B12b to learn whether she had a vitamin B12 dependency disorder. Immediately after the injection, her chest pain disappeared. When the pain returned two days later, I gave her another injection of B12b and again the pain disappeared. I then taught the patient how to give her own injections of the vitamin. For years now she has given herself an injection every few days. When she stops the injections, the chest pain returns.

Vitamin B12 is helping the chemistry of her heart muscle. Surely one injection did not make her coronary arteries larger.

I've seen patients with angina lose their pain when they took other nutrients. Magnesium, vitamin E, vitamin C, selenium, L-carnitine and other nutrients have stopped heart pains in my patients.

This is not surprising when you learn that breathing oxygen in strong concentrations stops most heart pain. The oxygen doesn't make arteries larger. It makes the chemistry of the heart muscle more efficient. If the heart lacks magnesium, for example, extra oxygen allows the heart muscle to use its subnormal amount of magnesium more efficiently.

It's the same when you toss a burning match into a bottle of oxygen. The fire flares because the oxygen speeds the chemical reaction.

Some cardiologists are beginning to agree with my point of view. They too suspect that food and environmental incompatibilities and the chemistry of the heart muscle, not the size of the arteries, cause most heart pain and heart attacks.

Running, by increasing the stress on the heart muscle, magnifies any chemical defects in the muscle. To illustrate, magnesium is commonly deficient in people eating the average American diet. The proper balance of calcium and magnesium is critically important for the functioning of the heart muscle. An improper balance strains the heart's chemistry. When people with low magnesium run, they magnify their chemical defect and risk trouble. *The stress of running when the heart muscle has an imperfect chemistry explains why runners too often drop dead while running.*

I should point out that as we get older our chemistry becomes less efficient. That's why athletes often reach their peak in their twenties and begin going downhill during their thirties. As body chemistry becomes less efficient, it's no longer able to make up for defects. If you have too little magnesium at age 20, it's less serious than a magnesium deficiency at age 40.

Statistics show that after a heart attack patients who take up running live longer than non-runners. Agreed, but only the less chemically damaged people feel good enough to run. Researchers don't put patients in "running" or "non-running" groups by random selection. Patients run only if they volunteer to run. If a patient's chemistry is dreadful and he feels nervous, exhausted, and depressed, he isn't likely to join the running group.

The running group is the healthier group, the less biochemically deficient group to start with. That—not the act of running—explains why they live longer.

How Much Walking? How Often?

By now the readers of this book realize there's no such thing as buying good health. You must get good health the old-fashioned way.

Of course, before starting any exercise program—even walking—you should consult your physician.

I advise most of my patients to begin walking as best they can. I ask them to work up gradually to an hour's walk every day, preferably during daylight hours so they'll get full-spectrum light. Regardless of physical condition, almost everyone can walk.

I have a patient paralyzed from spinal cord damage caused by a lack of vitamin B12. He arrived at my office in a wheelchair. With an arm to lean on, he now walks around the block and even climbs stairs.

I have another patient who spent most of her time in bed because of severe atrophic arthritis. With the help of a nurse, she now walks for 20 minutes a day.

If those two people can walk, you can walk.

Excuses

During the winter, patients tell me it's too cold to walk outside. Nonsense, it's never too cold for a walk. Eskimos walk during the winter. They simply dress for the cold. Wear long johns, heavy wool socks, a headpiece that covers your ears. Most important, cover your mouth and nose with heavy cotton. An old bath towel washed with baking soda is often the best choice. Mittens are warmer than gloves.

It's too hot to walk.
I'm hungry.
It's raining.
I'll walk later.
I'll walk twice as far tomorrow.
I don't want to live bad enough to walk.
I've earned a rest. I'm going to have a sandwich and a beer and
    watch the game on TV.
I don't believe that nonsense about work and walking.
I don't make any money walking.
I might get hit by a car. I'm safer in the house.
. . . and on and on the excuses flow . . .

Our natural inclination is to rest. Our minds automatically come up with "good" reasons for doing what we want to do.

Because walking will become a regular part of your life, you should buy proper clothes for it. Select loose clothes, warm clothes for winter and cool clothes for summer. Heavy all-cotton socks are especially important. Wash your socks with baking soda and hot water. If you need warmer socks for wintertime, wear thin white cottons socks beneath thick wool stocks.

Need I tell you not to wear your diamond necklace when you go for a walk? Yes, I do need to tell you. I've seen too many people in New York take chances.

I rarely see anyone wearing proper shoes. Apparently all shoe designers have narrow feet that end in delicate points.

Here's how to find a shoe that fits. With pencil in hand, place a large sheet of paper on the floor. Stand on the paper. Put your weight on your foot. Draw around the edges of your foot. Are you surprised that you have duck-shaped feet? Don't be upset. Queen Elizabeth and

David Rockefeller also have duck-shaped feet. A Mrs. Sweeney is the only person I know who doesn't have duck-shaped feet.

It's difficult to find a shoe shaped like your foot.

Clark's Wallabee shoes are inexpensive and a good solution, though they have crepe soles. (*When the surface you're walking on is damp or icy, never wear shoes with crepe soles.*)

There's another solution. Buy shoes that can easily assume the shape of your foot. Shoes should have either no heels or heels no more than half an inch. On city streets, rubber soles make walking more comfortable.

Do not buy a shoe that smells like a chemical factory!

THE CHIROPODIST

A few months ago a chiropodist consulted me. This man had spent his professional life trying to correct foot problems. He knew nothing about the importance of walking, or about nutrition. He thought he had a good workout after walking from the parking lot to a patient's room in the hospital. His idea of a well-balanced meal was wine, pizza, ice cream, and coffee. Among other suggestions, I asked him to start walking.

"I can't walk. My feet are too bad," was his reply.

I had him take off his shoes and walk to the door and back a few times.

True, he had inadequate feet. I've never seen a more slew-footed, flat-footed member of the human race. I examined his shoes. They had pointed toes, the style you would expect to see on a jazz trumpet player. They had heavy arch supports that looked and felt as if an iron foundry made them.

I drew an outline of his very duck-shaped foot and suggested a proper shoe.

"And leave out your arch supporters when you walk," I advised.

The man went pale and looked faint.

"I can't walk six blocks without arch supports," he sputtered. He began pulling on his shoes as if afraid I would confiscate his arch supports.

"Then walk six blocks. Every week add another block until you're walking an hour a day."

"I could never walk without my arch supports," he said. A few mintues later he fled my office and never returned. He's probably still suffering from his complaint. At least he still has his arch supports. He probably sleeps with them.

Back braces and arch supports are temporary measures. They support weakened parts of the body. They also make the trouble worse. Backs get weaker when supported. You cannot make arches stronger by supporting them. The answer is not support, but a proper diet and exercise, especially walking.

Braces and supports are usually a part of what I call the show biz of medicine.

How to Walk Correctly

If possible, walk with a free stride. Our primitive ancestors walked to go someplace, not to admire the flowers and the sunsets. Try to walk a full hour without stopping. I don't know about you, but I get some of my best ideas while walking.

What are the walking conditions in your town? Probably they're no rougher than here in Manhattan. In Los Angeles the rare person who walks is king. In L.A., cars startle me when they stop to let me cross a street. After visiting L.A. for a few days and returning to Manhattan, cars nearly run me down. Here the drivers are out to get you, not only automobile drivers, but the motor bikers and especially the bicyclists.

Fortunately for every attack, there's a defense. Your best defense in New York—aside from watching closely and jumping broadly—is an umbrella or a walking stick. When carried horizontally by your side, it should project two feet in front and behind you. Both bicyclists and motorists will respect such an instrument. Bicycle riders shudder at the thought of having a walking stick accidentally thrust between their spokes. Motorists don't want scratches on their car doors.

If you're walking in the city, if possible avoid the heaviest traffic. Early mornings are best. Sometimes you have no choice. Then at least walk up wind from the automobiles so you'll breathe as few fumes as possible. On close, warm, muggy days it's especially important to avoid heavy traffic.

Many people are allergic to plants and trees. They often do better on city streets. I've seen a few people who get reactions to tarmac on hot days.

How often should you walk? That's an easy one: every day.

How far? As far as you can make it in half an hour. Then turn around and head back for half an hour.

Your Teeth Need Exercise Too

Cavities are part of the Newbold Syndrome, diseases of civilization caused by eating modern foods.

Also part of the Newbold Syndrome: periodontal (gum) diseases and loss of bone mass in the jaw.

No matter how compatible the food you eat is with your body chemistry and no matter how perfect your nutritional supplements might be, they will not help unless your teeth have vigorous exercise.

How do you exercise teeth?

You do not exercise teeth by eating rice, eggs, potatoes, hamburgers, or chocolate ice cream.

You exercise your back teeth by eating tough meat. The tougher the better.

How do you exercise front teeth?

There's only one way: pick meat up with your hands and bite off chunks. If need be, also pull and tear at the meat. (In most quarters it's considered bad table manners to growl when you do this!)

The next time you dine at the Ritz, explain to Henri, the maitre d', that you are a patient of Dr. Newbold and he requires you to eat with your fingers. If Henri gives you a supercilious look, get back at him. Next time order your steak boiled medium in Perrier water!

The Secret

In the first chapter I promised to hide an important tip on losing weight in one of the later chapters. Here's the tip, a tip discovered by me and known only to me: If you eat all of your food with your fingers, you will lose weight much faster. Why? It will take less food to satisfy you. I discovered this quite by chance when trying to devise ways to exercise the front teeth.

Years ago I had dinner in London at the home of Lord and Lady Clwyd. For dessert we were served an apple, a plain apple sitting in a saucer in half an inch of water. The other people at the table cut a wedge from the apple, ate it, cut another, ate it, and so on.

I took my apple from the water, peeled it, then proceeded—horse-like—to take noisy bites of the apple. Several people glanced at the ugly American.

I smiled and said, "I say, didn't any of your nannies teach you how to eat an apple properly?"

I wanted to give them a lecture on English teeth, the worst in the world, but restrained myself.

Actress Ellen Burstyn is the only one who ever invited me back for a second meal.

Exercises Other Than Walking

Even though every form of activity is desirable, no exercise takes the place of walking.

Swimming in chlorinated water may irritate your nose, throat, or lungs. The odor of chlorine sends some people on eating sprees. We've already discussed the drawbacks of running. Tennis and handball make for good workouts. Weight-lifting is great, but by itself is inadequate. The Royal Canadian Air Force Exercise Plan for Physical Fitness takes only 12 or 13 minutes a day. It has a very well graduated program that's suitable for most people. The Air Force exercises plus weight-lifting plus walking is an ideal combination.

Walking, however, is where it's at. After a short time, walking is easier. It becomes a part of your routine life. Only when we change our routine is it difficult. Within a month, you won't want to *stop* walking. After a good walk, you'll feel the pleasant difference in your body. Something "tells us" that walking improves our body chemistry.

Walk in the morning, walk at noon, walk after lunch, walk at night. Walk as much as you can. If you can't walk, crawl!

Why did they make our brains so short and our legs so long? Answer: For survival. Our legs are more important than our brains.

23

If You Fail to Lose Weight

The world belongs to the meat eater, and sometimes you got to eat it raw.

—WILLIAM FAULKNER

Let's get through this one in a hurry so you can read Chapter 25, the chapter you've been looking forward to, the chapter called "How to Cheat and Stay Slender." If you're discouraged because you seem to be at an impasse or plateau and can't seem to lose any more weight, check your habits against the factors below to see where you've gone wrong.

Alcohol: Sorry, but you cannot drink and lose weight.

Browned and Burned: Remember not to eat any browned or burned meat or fat. Not only will it give some people cancer and make them feel bad, but often it makes people hungry.

Cheating: Don't cheat until you've reached your goal. If you're cheating and not losing two to three pounds a week, stop cheating entirely. You'll fail at this weight losing game.

Cold: If you're doing everything right and not losing, put one or more meals in the refrigerator and chill it after cooking. Then eat it cold.

Cooking: Remember, cook with electricity, not with gas. Gas may make you hungry and may give you cancer. Otherwise cooking with gas is great—unless you have asthma, lupus, arthritis, abdominal discomfort and a host of other troubles.

196

Drinks: "Diet" sodas commonly knock out the appestat center and make people hungry. Same for coffee, tea, herbal teas—and all other drinks. Even the wrong water can make you hungry.

Drugs: Cocaine, opium, heroin and such heavy duty drugs will help you lose weight, but they will do a number on your head and on your life. Don't do them. On proper nutritional supplements and a proper diet, most people lose interest in them.

Environment: If you keep going off your diet, maybe something in your environment is knocking out your appestat. Reread Chapter 11. Cut off the gas. Cook only with electricity? Do you have a cat? Does a close relative or your best friend have a cat? Make up? Hair dye? Copy machine at work? Plants or fluorescent lighting at work?

Exercise: If you are not losing two to three pounds a week, maybe you aren't walking an hour and five mintues a day. Maybe you're "trying to walk" or maybe you're breaking your walk up into two 30-minute periods. You need to walk every day including Sunday. A stroll with a child won't do. You've got to walk like you mean it.

Fear: When some people find themselves losing weight it frightens them. I suppose it's a fear that goes back to our cave man days when we feared starvation. I've helped a number of people lose weight. None of them starved.

Some women fear that if they lose weight they'll become too attractive to men and complications will arise. Only once in my practice did this actually happen. She learned how to manage the problem.

Frequency: Often people think the earth will open up at their feet and something horrible will happen to them unless they eat three times a day. Not true—unless they are addicted to a food and feel withdrawal symptoms unless they eat that food frequently. The solution to that problem is to get off the food to which they're addicted. Most people on a high meat and a little vegetable diet only need to eat twice a day. Try eating twice a day.

Fruit: Fruit can defeat you, especially after your weight begins coming down out of the stratosphere. If you aren't losing properly, cut down on your fruit. If it makes you hungry, or if you still aren't losing, cut all fruit from your diet. After four or five days you'll hardly miss it.

Hands: If you're doing everything right and still not losing, pick your meat up in your hands, bite off chunks and eat it. Why, I don't know, but it's impossible to eat as much if you renounce the knife and fork.

Hormones: Sex hormones, birth control pills and adrenal cortical steroid hormones may keep you from losing weight.

Nutritional supplements: Test your vitamins, minerals and unsaturated fats by having them one at a time to learn whether you've developed an incompatibility to one of them that knocks out your appestat and makes you spree eat.

Plateaus: Now and then you'll hit plateaus where your weight stays the same. Hang on. If you're doing everything right, your weight *will* start plunging again.

Pot: You can't smoke pot and lose weight.

Seasoning: Don't season food. Seasoning will make you hungry and make you eat more. Cows like salt. Lions—like you—do without it very well.

Tranquilizers, sleeping pills and antidepressants: They may defeat your weight loss program. After you're on proper nutritional supplements and a proper diet, you probably won't need them.

Vegetables: Stay with no more than half a cup per meal. Remember, no beans, peas, root vegetables such as carrots, potatoes, parsnips and turnips. Always eat your vegetables raw. Many people find some vegetables that are incompatible with their chemistry. If it's incompatible, even lettuce can knock out your appestat and send you on an eating spree. In truth, lettuce frequently does. Calories have nothing to do with the problem.

If nothing else works: What I've outlined has always worked for my patients. If you fail to lose weight, eat with your fingers and eat all of your food cold.

Remember, the world really is out to get you.

If You Cheat and Can't Get Back on Your Diet

First get your physician's approval, then. . . . Stuff yourself with the foods you're cheating with. For example, if you're cheating with chocolate ice cream, eat a quart of chocolate ice cream, then another quart, then another and if possible even more, until you throw up.

After gorging yourself, then fast for four days. Eat nothing at all for four days. Have nothing but water to drink.

Be careful while fasting. Do not drive a car or engage in dangerous activity such as using an electric saw. If you go out of the house, have someone go with you. If you feel weak, lie down.

You will read all sorts of nonsense about how to end a fast with fruit juices, etc. To end a fast, you simply start eating again. There's only one precaution: Be careful not to overeat. Go back on your diet and this time stay on it.

Persistence is the horse that wins.

24

After Reaching Your Goal

The best laid schemes o' mice and men
Gang aft a-gley.

—ROBERT BURNS

IAN MARKS

Wearing a green suit when he first visited me on St. Patrick's Day, Ian Marks looked like a gift-wrapped man mountain at 383 pounds. A jovial beer-tipsy hail-fellow, he didn't impress me as a man who would stick to a project such as losing weight. To my surprise, he cooperated very well. Under my program his weight plunged to 197 pounds.

Incidentally, his serum cholesterol fell from 278 to 188, while his triglycerides went from 165 to 69, and his fasting blood sugar changed from 118 to 93. At the same time his HDL (the "good" type of fat in the blood) climbed from 35 (13 percent) to 58 (30 percent).

"This is the most critical phase of weight loss," I told him once he had reached his goal. "For the next six months, you'll be living through a very dangerous time."

Ian was full of confidence and quite cocky, as people tend to be after accomplishing a great feat. Nothing would go wrong. He had learned his lesson. He would never be fat again.

"I want to see you every two weeks until I'm satisfied that your weight will remain stable."

Impossible. He was going to Japan for a tour and then would visit friends for a few weeks. He would call for an appointment in a couple of months.

"I don't feel good about this," I told him.

"Not to worry. I'm on top of this weight thing."

Problems

Three months later, Ian Marks—50 pounds heavier—visited my office. In Japan, beef rib steaks and veal chops, the two foods that had formed the backbone of Ian's weight-loss diet, sold for $40 a pound. He had tried to make do on fish and rice. It hadn't worked. Those foods made him not only hungry, but depressed and tense. When he returned to the States, he tried to come off rice, but had withdrawal symptoms. He misinterpreted them and thought he was having emotional problems.

Ian visited a psychologist who convinced him that all of his troubles came from a troubled childhood. Food incompatibilities were not his real problem.

Depressed people become emotionally dependent. Because going off his diet exposed Ian to foods that he couldn't tolerate and left him depressed, Ian quickly became emotionally dependent upon the psychologist.

"Look, just get back on your diet," I told Ian. "You'll have withdrawal symptoms for a few days, then your 'psychological problems' will vanish and your weight will go back down again."

"I don't know about that. . . ."

"I do. Let's play a game. Let's pretend that I know more about weight reduction and nutrition than either you or your psychologist. Probably I know more about psychology, too. I'm a qualified psychiatrist. I was on the faculty teaching psychiatry at Northwestern University School of Medicine. Also, I wrote a textbook on psychology that's used in universities around the world."

"Let me think about it."

When Ian left for Japan, I thought he was lost. Now I knew he was lost.

Six Months Later

Ian returned to see me only one more time. He had gained 81 pounds. He was being brainwashed by his psychologist, who kept telling Ian that his weight problems were emotional in origin, that they would go away once he "solved his emotional problems."

No amount of reasoning would get Ian back on his diet.

One of his friends told me a year later that Ian was close to his former size. People are infinitely creative when it comes to finding ways to fail at losing weight and keeping it off.

I'm happy to report that Ian's failure was an exception. Most of my patients keep their slender figures. It seems that I have talked a great deal about my failures. It's because I want you to learn from them.

Your Ideal Weight

Most books on dieting fill up the last half with meaningless tables showing the vitamin/mineral/caloric values of foods. Also, they have tables showing your "ideal weight." Here you'll find no such tables and charts. Today, no one knows what vitamins and minerals are in foods. If you want dependable vitamins and minerals, take them as outlined in this book. Some farmers grow foods in such bizarre ways we can no longer depend upon foods to supply vitamins and minerals.

Are you at your correct weight?

"Dr. Newbold, my face is so thin!" Many women look at themselves in the mirror, observe how much padding they have left in their faces and try to judge whether they've lost enough weight. That's not the way to judge proper weight.

"Dr. Newbold, I can see my ribs!" Women worry when they look at themselves in the mirror and see their ribs. You *should* see your ribs! The trouble is that in our too-plump society, women haven't seen their ribs in so long they've forgotten how they look. Instead of seeing themselves as sleek and fashionable, they think they're close to starving to death. Not so. If you have doubts, study the models in fashion magazines.

Not long ago Regis Philbin interviewed me on a TV talk show. Models in a fashion show went on before me. After my interview, the models were to return for the second part of the fashion parade. At the edge of the room—out of camera range—it amazed me to see a group of models changing into the evening gowns they were about to display. The models wore panty hose, shoes and nothing else. I assure you that they were slender, svelte, fashionable—and their ribs showed.

Some women, I've come to learn over the years, complain that they're too thin over their chests when they mean that their breasts aren't as large as before. True, overweight women usually have fuller breasts.

In my view, staying fat is not the way to keep breasts full. Remember, overweight women develop cancer of the breast more often than do their slender sisters. Better some than none—and sophisticated men know that women with small breasts are more desirable: They try harder!

(Is that a sexist statement? I can hide my masculine anatomy by wearing trousers, but I cannot hide my masculine mind. Love me or leave me.)

The Newbold Test for Women

Forget about weight charts and the scales. Make what I call the "Newbold Test."

Stand barefooted and nude on the floor. Face a mirror. Using your thumbs and the index fingers of both hands, take a big pinch of the fat over your upper, outer thighs. Are you able to pinch fat? If you find a fat pad, you aren't at your ideal weight.

On most women the fat over the upper outer thighs is the last to go.

A small percentage of women with thin thighs must pinch for fat over their abdomens.

In primitive times, overweight persons could better withstand the foodless days they had to endure. Those of us in the western world no longer face foodless days. We don't need fat in the bank.

The Newbold Test for Men

Women pinch their thighs. Men pinch their abdomens. If you're an overweight man and stand nude to face a mirror, you may see a bulge of fat on each side of your waist. If you pinch, you pick up fat.

Now use your pinching fingers to test for fat about two inches to the side of your navel. Now you know whether you need to lose more weight.

Men worry when they lose weight because they feel they're getting smaller. Mistakenly, they equate sheer size—including fat—as a measure of their power.

Recently I had an asthmatic as a patient. As we removed the foods to which he was allergic, the foods that caused his asthma, he quite naturally lost excess weight. Because he was a weight lifter and body-builder, he nearly panicked. He was certain he was going to end up so thin the other men at the gym would laugh at him.

As it turned out, as he lost fat, he gained definition in his muscles. In other words, his individual muscles stood out more sharply than before. Instead of laughing at him, the other men began asking what he was eating to bring about such great definition.

Don't Worry! You won't become too thin on this diet. On this diet I've repeatedly seen thin people gain weight.

I wish I could tell you that after reaching your proper weight you could eat apple pie à la mode and chocolate bonbons as often as you like and still keep your stylish figure.

After following most diets, only one percent of the people who lose weight keep it off. We no longer live in a jungle where grizzly bears and saber-toothed tigers wait behind a bush to pounce upon us. The great hunters from the tribe on the other side of the mountain are no longer likely to run us through with spears and drag away our mates. Today we're threatened by the neon-flashing signs above ice cream parlors, by TV commercials that show drippingly tempting sugary desserts, and by the supermarket where we must pass by the gooey goodies to reach the mundane things like the meats and vegetables.

From sea to shining sea, bright, aggressive men are sitting around boardroom tables trying to decide how best to transfer the money from your pockets into their pockets. They add sugar to canned vegetables because they know you'll buy more of them if they're sweet. They employ scientists to create new chemicals to add to soft drinks to make their color and their tastes irresistible. They hire admen to photograph dancing girls so you'll equate carbohydrate-rich foods with sex and social status. Believe me, the world is still populated with saber-toothed tigers and spear-throwing natives that are out to get you. They've just gone modern and wear clever disguises.

If possible, stay on your diet. Don't let the men who ride around in chauffeured limousines get their hands into your pockets.

Once You Reach Ideal Weight

You can be a bit more liberal with your fruits. Many people can tolerate up to a cup of fresh raw fruit once a day. Eat one fruit at a time. Do not repeat the fruit for 72 hours. That way you will learn which fruits agree with you and which do not.

- ◆ Peel what you can and wash what you cannot peel.
- ◆ Many people do not tolerate mangoes, red delicious apples, pineapples, grapes, bananas and oranges. Avoid them until you learn more about basics. Then test them.
- ◆ Never have fruit juice or dried fruit. Dried fruits are full of sprays, preservatives and molds. People react poorly to dried fruit.
- ◆ Both juices and dried fruits have concentrated carbohydrates. Even ex-overweight people can't handle them.

Carbohydrates, not fats, are your enemies.

Being Human . . .

Sooner or later you'll cheat.

If possible, stay on the straight and narrow. If, on the other hand, come what may, you're determined to cheat, read the next chapter—and learn how to do it properly.

The Duchess of Windsor said it for the modern women, "You can't be too rich or too thin."

Don't read the next chapter until you've reached your ideal weight!

25

How to Cheat and Stay Slender

Better stay with nurse,
You might find something worse.

To Lie or Not to Lie?

I'm not naive. I know that fortunes have been made selling books that tell people how to lose weight. If I were seeking a fortune, I'd tell you what you want to hear. I'd give you a pseudo-scientific explanation about why it worked, then I'd advise something like: Sprinkle half a teaspoon of dried kumquat rinds on your food once a day, and you can eat all the pasta and chocolate mousse you want. The pounds and inches will melt away.

Look, Mozart knew what he was doing was right. Even if the emperor thought Mozart's music had "too many notes," Mozart knew he was right. He could have written music to please, like Salieri, and could have made enough money to live like a prince. Money wasn't what Mozart wanted. He wanted something far more valuable than money.

So do I.

Mind you, I'm not opposed to making money, but any Salieri can please the people and the powers that be and make money—and have his work die with his flesh.

So, here goes . . . more truths, truths that you hoped not to hear.

Danger!

Do you think it would be dangerous for you to put on boxing gloves and climb into the ring to fight 12 rounds with Iron Mike Tyson? That's child's play compared to the dangers that lurk in the dark world of diet cheating.

What do you say about this scenario: You become addicted to heroin. You're hospitalized for three months for detoxification and rehabilitation. After returning to your family and going back to work, you visit your doctor and say, "Say Doc, what do you think about my doing a little heroin only on Saturday nights?"

Almost any doctor would say, "You can't handle heroin. You'll become addicted again and be back in the heroin awfuls so fast you'll think a tornado hit you."

And what if you just graduated from rehab after coming off cocaine and wanted to do just a few pipes?

And if you had a history of going on six-week drinking sprees and had been an abstaining member of AA for five years and asked about having a few drinks to celebrate your sobriety—"Just one drink every five years, Doc. Is that unreasonable?"

I know you don't believe me, but I kid you not. Grains (especially wheat) and table sugar are 10 times as addictive as heroin, cocaine and alcohol combined.

Grains and table sugar (and milk and milk products are almost as bad) are even more dangerous than alcohol, cocaine and heroin because they're inexpensive, relatively socially acceptable, and many of your friends are addicted to them.

Cheating is always extremely dangerous, especially after losing weight. Advising people not to cheat, however, is like advising abstinence for birth control. In the practical world, people won't listen.

Please don't quote me as saying that once you lose weight, you're free to cheat. If you're determined to cheat, however, you need to know how to cheat and escape with the least possible damage. Certainly cheating is not for amateurs.

I've written this chapter to help people who are going to cheat, to cheat scientifically.

Why Do We Like to Cheat?

It was the ambitious, the adventurous, the creative, the bored who left their comfortable homelands and sailed to America. They conquered and tamed a wild land, built farms and factories and skyscrapers. Such people don't take easily to the yoke of civilization. Today we're no different from our musket-shooting, knife-wielding, cement-pouring ancestors who struggled to build a great civilization.

If we are busy with primitive, physical activities—following a mule and a plow, sewing clothes and cooking for our six children, or driving a covered wagon to California—we have little interest in cheating. Let that same frontiersperson move into a Fifth Avenue apartment with running water, a microwave oven, and a 40-hour-a-week desk job, and that person will be ready to cheat—if only to drive away the wolves of boredom.

Civilization—and living in groups of more than 30 people—is a great threat to us, and we are far from learning how to handle it. Certainly evolution has not yet molded our biochemistry to handle civilization with grace.

First, ask yourself why you feel compelled to cheat. Often the desire to cheat means that something knocked out your appestat center, something such as perfume, or the neighbor's cat. Even innocent-appearing fruit is a common trigger. Try very hard to identify what hit you. Change things in your diet and your environment until you discover the trouble maker.

The second most common cause of cheating is a withdrawal reaction. If you become addicted to a food again and don't eat that food, you'll have cravings for carbohydrates for four days. The easiest way to handle the problem is to go on a four-day water fast.

You might cheat simply because you're hungry. See number 10 in the list that follows.

Guidelines for Cheating

1. After finishing in the bathroom, weigh yourself first thing every morning. Tape a piece of paper to the wall beside the scales and write down your weight. Don't allow your weight to creep up. Regaining 150 pounds starts with one, two and then three pounds.

You must make choices. What do you want, a car that will tear away at the first hint of the green light and reach 60 miles per hour in six seconds, or do you want a car that will travel 30 miles on a gallon of gas?

Either stay close to your diet—or get fat again. Now that you've read this book and learned how to stay slender, you have no excuse except lack of choice.

2. If you've got to cheat, cheat with fruit. You can only eat so much fruit before you'll get diarrhea.

3. If you're going to cheat simply because you've decided you want the forbidden, confine your cheating to one time a week. The biggest problem with cheating is becoming readdicted to foods that are incompatible with your biochemistry. If you cheat only once a week, you won't become addicted. If you cheat twice a week, you'll almost surely get addicted again and put weight back on.

4. If you cheat twice a week and become addicted, a four- or five-day water fast is the best way to break the addiction (with your physician's approval).

5. If you gain five pounds, go on a five-day water fast, not to lose weight but to escape the addiction (with your physician's approval).

6. If you're going to cheat by drinking alcoholic beverages, and if you're determined also to cheat by eating forbidden foods, do your food cheat with your drink cheat.

7. If you're going to cheat with alcohol, a non-grain-based alcohol is usually best. That means no beer, whiskey, gin or vodka. If pressed to the wall, I will admit that of those mentioned, gin is usually best tolerated. If you are not sensitive to potatoes, a potato-based vodka is available and is the best tolerated vodka.

If you're going to cheat with alcohol, the least harmful is French champagne, brut. To many people's surprise, "brut" champagne is less sweet than the "extra dry." Not only is brut French champagne low in carbohydrates, but it's expensive, so you're less likely to become addicted to it. It tends to be more compatible with more people's chemistry—and at least you'll be cheating with class!

Next best choice is light dry white wines. Most people tolerate inexpensive wines better than expensive wines, probably because they have fewer chemicals such as aldehydes that form during aging. At the moment, choose Almaden Mountain Chablis or Gallo's Sauvignon Blanc. Careful: They might change the formula next week.

Of the stronger alcoholic drinks, cognac or calvados—a brandy made from fermented apples—is a reasonable bet. They're better tolerated than whiskeys, which have traces of grains in them. Today even most vodkas contain grains.

Casanova knew that morals and good resolutions were soluble in alcohol. One of the big problems with drinking alcohol is, after a glass or two you're likely to say, "To hell with Newbold and his damned diet! I'm going to eat whatever I want to!" Or you might say, "I'm not fat any longer. I can eat whatever I want to." Or, "I've conquered my eating problems." Or, "I'll go back on my diet tomorrow." Then you dig into a monumental cheat.

8. If you must cheat, *rotate your cheats!* I can't stress that too much. If on Christmas Day you cheat by drinking calvados, make your New Year's Eve cheat champagne. If you should ever become foolish enough to cheat by eating cake, make your next absolutely forbidden cheat sherbet.

9. Try never to cheat with foods that contain grains or table sugar. Wheat is dangerous. Sugar ranks second. If you do cheat, cheat with a food that contains much fat. I know that's contrary to everything you hear or read. But you heard me correctly. Believe me, I know more about the subject than other "authorities." The fat fills you up and limits the cheat. Also, fat slows the entrance of other foods into your body so your chemistry can adjust to them better.

10. Sometimes people cheat simply because they're hungry. Be sure you're eating enough fat. Only fats and carbohydrates will satisfy your caloric needs. Fats have more than two times as many calories as carbohydrates, but they satisfy four or five times as much.

Fish and chicken do not have much fat. People who eat fish or chicken are often hungry. Their hunger may drive them to cheat. People who eat mostly beef rib steaks feel satisfied and are less likely to cheat.

Remember: If you eat the beef fat, take your vitamins, minerals and oils. Stay off grains, milk products, table sugar and nuts. Your cholesterol will go down and your HDL ("good" fats) will go up.

If you walk for an hour each day, it helps even more. There's no substitute for walking.

Remember: *Do not eat burned or browned fats, or fats cooked with gas.*

11. If you're going to cheat, cheat before you eat—then don't eat.
12. If you're going to cheat, you'll react less if you take two Bufferin tablets 30 minutes before.
13. Vitamin B6 (200 to 1200 mg), vitamin C (4,000 to 8,000 mg), dolomite powder (one teaspoon), L-carnitine (500 mg), and vitamin B12 (1,000 to 6,000 mcg by injection) before a cheat often reduce reactions. Alka-Seltzer Gold also helps both before and after. These items mentioned help reduce the severity of withdrawal reactions. (Do not take anything without your physican's approval.)

If taken before you cheat, the above will often help reduce your desire to cheat.

14. To stay slender you must devleop new activities to fill the void left by not eating. Play golf or get an evening job or walk to Timbuktu—anything as long as it helps take up the slack. Physical activity is best.
15. Cheat only *after* you've reached your ideal weight.

In the practical world of everyday life, people who lose weight start cheating. After a certain time—or after a certain number of gained pounds—most of my patients realize what's happening and have a talk with themselves and stop cheating.

Remember that 95 percent of our brains are used 97 percent of the time finding "logical" reasons for doing what we want to do. When the minister's single daughter gets pregnant, she tells her father, "It felt so good, I thought God wanted me to."

Is Dr. Newbold a great and noble person? You can hear arguments both ways on that question. One thing is certain: I am not a great and noble person when it comes to eating. I stay on my diet—or cheat very carefully and scientifically—for several purely selfish reasons.

1. I feel bad when I cheat.
2. My brain will not work well when I cheat.

3. I know it will kill me if my cheating gets out of hand.

You want to improve your appearance, to feel great, to have your brain work at its best—and to live a long, productive life. Now you know the secrets.

And every day of your life remember. . . .

All of us—poor man, rich man, beggar man, thief—are dancing to a tune played by evolution.

Appendix

Animal Fat and Cancer of the Colon
Letter to the *New England Journal Of Medicine*

Arnold S. Relman, M.D., Editor-in-Chief
New England Journal of Medicine
10 Shattuck Street
Boston MA 02115
December 15, 1990

Dear Dr. Relman:

The December 13, 1990 article in the *New England Journal of Medicine* by Willet is fatally flawed and did not lead to the conclusion that eating red meat might increase the risk of colon cancer. Here are the paper's 16 greatest flaws:

1. No distinction between eating preserved meat (bacon with carcinogenic nitrites and carcinogenic smoked meats) and fresh meat.
2. No distinction between aged and unaged meat. Aged meat has more oxidized fat. Oxidized fat is carcinogenic.
3. No mention of the thickness of the meat. Ground and thinly cut meat has more oxidized fat per gram.
4. Was the meat boiled, broiled, pan fried? The carcinogenicity of browned meat is famous.
5. Was it eaten cooked or raw (steak tartare)? Grinding meat increases oxidation, but eating it raw decreases exposure to oxidized fat.
6. Was meat reheated? Reheating increases oxidation.
7. Was the meat refrigerated? A roast eaten over days gives more oxidized fat.
8. Was the meat frozen? Freezing alters its chemistry.
9. Various cuts of meat taste different, hence must be chemically different. Possibly different cuts react in the bowel in different ways.

213

10. Was the burned and browned meat and fat discarded?

11. What type of heat was used for cooking? Meat cooked over gas or in gas ovens takes up hydrocarbons, thus becomes carcinogenic.

12. Because vitamin A, beta carotene, vitamin C, calcium, selenium, etc. are protective against cancer, we need the levels of such nutrients in those studied.

13. No mention of breed of animals or what the animals were fed. Breed, feed and physical activity alter the chemistry of meat.

14. Was the meat cryovaced? Cryovacing alters the chemistry of meat.

15. People eating little meat (like the nurses eating red meat once a month) take more vitamins, drink little alcohol, buy cheap cuts of meats, do not refrigerate meat.

16. Were the subjects black or white? They metabolize meat differently.[1]

If Willet had fed each group 1¼ inch thick, medium boiled, fresh beef mid-rib rib steak from penned, corn-fed Aberdeen Angus cattle, would he have found any difference in the cancer rates between nurses eating red meat daily and those eating it only once a month? Probably not.

The fault, dear Willet, lies in the way we process and cook meat, and the food and drink we take with meat, not in meat itself. Not only does fat, like roughage, facilitate bowel transit, but, following certain guidelines, eating fatty red meat lowers cholesterol and raises HDL.[2-14]

1. Edozien J. (Professor of Nutrition, University of North Carolina) Personal communication 2–21–89.

2. Lieb CW. The effects on human beings of a twelve months' exclusive meat diet. JAMA 1929; 93:20–21.

3. Newbold HL. The reduction of serum cholesterol while feeding a high animal fat diet. International Journal for Vitamin and Nutrition Research 1986; 56:190.

4. Newbold HL. Reducing Serum Cholesterol by Feeding a High Animal Fat Diet. Southern Medical Journal 1988; 81:61–63.

Reply to the above letter to the *New England Journal of Medicine*

THE NEW ENGLAND JOURNAL OF MEDICINE

10 Shattuck Street, Boston, Massachusetts 02115-6094
—Telephone 617/734-9800

Editorial Offices

Correspondence No. 90-3829   February 15, 1991

H. L. Newbold M.D.
115 East 34th Street
New York NY 10016

Dear Dr. Newbold:

Your letter referring to the Willet Original Article of December 13 has been received. Because of the limited availability of space we can publish only a fraction of the letters we receive. Although we will not be able to print yours, we have forwarded a copy to the authors in case they wish to reply directly to you.

Thank your for your interest in the *Journal.*

Sincerely yours,
Marcia Angell M.D.
Executive Editor

MEA/pml

Comment about the above letter

I dare say it was not lack of space that kept them from publishing the letter. They did not publish it because it made the editor appear poorly informed for accepting Willet's paper for publication.

H. L. Newbold, M. D.

References

Professional Publications by the Author

Newbold, H. L., Relationship between spontaneous allergic conditions and ascorbic acid, *Journal of Allergy*, vol.15: 385-88, Nov. 1944.

Newbold, H. L., Neurodermatitis, *Journal of the American Medical Association*, vol. 132, no. 11:674, Nov. 16, 1946.

Newbold, H. L., et al., Aneurysm of the left ventricle secondary to myocardial infarction, *Southern Medical Journal*, April 1949.

Newbold, H. L., et al., The use of chlorpromazine in psychotherapy, *Journal of Nervous and Mental Diseases*, March 1956.

Book: Newbold, H. L., and Steed, W. D., The use of chlorpromazine in psychotherapy. In *The New Chemotherapy in Mental Illness*, ed. by H. L. Gordon, Philosophical Library, New York 1958.

Newbold, H. L., Reduction of EST-induced fractures by the use of sodium pentobarbital and succinylcholine, *Diseases of the Nervous System*, vol. 19, no. 9:385-87, Sept. 1958.

Newbold, H. L., How one psychiatrist began using niacin, *Schizophrenia*, vol, 2, no. 4:150-60, 1970.

Book: Newbold, H. L., *The Psychiatric Programming of People*, Pergamon Press, New York 1972.

Newbold, H. L., The use of vitamin B-12b in psychiatric practice, *Journal of Orthomolecular Psychiatry*, vol. 1, no. 1, 1972.

Newbold, H. L., et al., Psychiatric syndromes produced by allergies: ecologic mental illness, *Journal of Orthomolecular Psychiatry*, vol. 2, no. 3, 1973.

Book: Newbold, H. L., *Mega-Nutrients for Your Nerves*, Wyden Books, New York, 1975. (Pocket size: Berkley)

Book: Newbold, H. L., *Doctor Newbold's Revolutionary New Discoveries About Weight Loss, How to master the hidden allergies that make you fat*, Rawson, New York, 1977. (Pocket size: NAL)

Book: Newbold, H. L., The use of B12 in psychiatric practice. In *Physician's Handbook on Orthomolecular Medicine*, ed. by Roger J. Williams and Dwight K. Kalita, Pergamon Press, New York, 1977.

Book: Newbold, H. L., *Vitamin C Against Cancer*, Stein and Day, New York, 1979. (Trade paperback and pocket size by Stein and Day.)

Newbold, H. L., The reduction of serum cholesterol while feeding a high animal fat diet, *International Journal for Vitamin and Nutrition Research*, vol. 56, no. 2:190, 1986.

Book: Newbold, H. L., *Mega-Nutrients*, The Body Press, Los Angeles, 1987.

Newbold, H. L., The medical origins of Duke University, *Southern Medical Journal*, vol. 80:799, June 1987.

Newbold, H. L., Reducing Serum Cholesterol by Feeding a High Animal Fat Diet, *Southern Medical Journal*, p. 61-63, Jan. 1988.

Newbold, H. L., Vitamin B-12, megaloblastic madness, and the founding of Duke University, *Medical Hypotheses*, p. 231-240, Nov. 1988.

Newbold, H. L., Vitamin B-12: placebo or neglected therapeutic tool? *Medical Hypotheses*, p. 155-164, March 1989.

Newbold, H. L., Nystatin for treatment of acne vulgaris, *Journal of the American Academy of Dermatology*, p. 861, May 1989.

Newbold, H. L., Vitamin B-12b as an antidote for over-sedation, *Medical Hypotheses*, vol. 30, no. 1, Sept. 1989.

Newbold, H. L., Dependence on vitamin B-12 injections, *Journal of the American Medical Association*, p. 1468, September 15, 1989.

Book: Newbold, H. L., *Dr. Newbold's Type-A/Type-B Weight Loss Book*, Keats, New Canaan 1991.

Book: Newbold, H. L., Reducing the Blacks' Disadvantages in a White-Designed Ecosystem. Completed. Submitted.

Book: Newbold, H. L., *Nutrition For Your Nerves*, Keats, New Canaan, 1992.

Book: Newbold, H. L., *The Newbold Syndrome: How to Cure The Incurable*. Completed.

Book: Newbold, H. L., *Dr. Newbold's How to Cure Diabetes Book*. Completed.

Other References

American Cancer Society, News Letter, p. 1, 3, Spring 1986.

Anand, B. K. and Brobeck J. R., Localization of a "feeding center" in the hypothalamus of the rat, *Proc. Soc. Exp. Biol. Med.*, 77:323, 1951.

Ardrey, R., *The Hunting Hypothesis*, Atheneum, New York, 1976.

Barnes, B. O., et al., *Heart Attack Rareness in Thyroid-Treated Patients*, Charles C. Thomas Co., Springfield, 1972.

Barnes, B. O., Basal temperature versus basal metabolism, *Journal of the American Medical Association*, 119:1072, August 1942.

Borum, P. R., and Fischer, K. D. (eds.), *Health Effects of Dietary Carnitine*, Life Sciences Research Office, Federation of American Society for Experimental Biology, Bethesda, 1983.

Brecher and Waxler, *Proc. Soc. Exp. Biol. Med.*, 70:498, 1949.

Brooks, C. M., et al., Experimental production of obesity in the monkey (Macaca Mulatta), *Fed. Proc.*, 1:11, 1942.

Brothwell D., Brothwell P., *Food in Antiquity*, Praeger Publishers, Inc., New York, 1969.

Brown, R., Ramirez, D., Taub, J., *The Physician and Sports Medicine*, 6:34-45, 1978.

Bryant, V. M., Jr., et al., The coprolites of man, *Scientific American*, Jan., 1975.

Carlson, A. J., *The Control of Hunger in Health and Disease*, University of Chicago Press, Chicago, 1914.

Coca, A. F., *The Pulse Test*, Arco Publishing Co., New York, 1972.

Cohen, M. N., *The Food Crisis in Prehistory*, Yale University Press, New Haven and London, 1977.

Congressional Record, United States of America, Proceedings and debates of the 94th congress, second session, vol. 122, no. 125, Aug. 24, 1976.

Correa, P., et al., Dietary determinants of gastric cancer in south Louisiana inhabitants, *JNCI*, 75:645-54, Oct. 1985.

Crawford, M., and Crawford, S., *What We Eat Today*, Spearman, London, 1972.

Delgado, J. M. R. and Anand, B. K., Increase in food intake induced by electrical stimulation of the lateral hypothalamus, *Am. J. Physiol.*, 172:162, 1953.

Dickey, L. D., ed., *Clinical Ecology*, Charles C. Thomas, Springfield, 1976.

DiSorbo, D. M., In vivo and in vitro inhibition of B16 melanoma growth by vitamin B6, *Nutr. Cancer*, 7:43-52, Jan.-June 1985.

Dohan, F. C., Cereals and schizophrenia, data and hypothesis, *Acta Psychiat. Scand.*, 42:125, 1968.

Dohan, F. C., Grasberg, J., Lowell, F., Johnson, H., and Arbegast, A. W., Cereal-free diet in relapsed schizophrenics, *Fed. Proc.*, 27:2, 1968.

Fischer, S., and Weber, P. C., *Nature*, 307:165-68, 1984.

Folkins, C., Lynch, S., and Gardner, M., *Archives of Physical Medicine and Rehabilitation*, 53:503-8, 1972.

Foran, J. A., Glenn, B. S., Silverman, W. Increased fish consumption may be risky, *Journal of the American Medical Association*, vol. 262, no. 1:28, July 7, 1989.

Foran, J. A., Cox, M., Croxton, D. Sport fish consumption advisories and projected cancer risk in the Great Lakes basin, *Am. J. Public Health*, 79:322-325, 1989.

Foulds, W. S., et al., *Lancet*, p. 35, Jan. 3, 1970.

Friedman, M. A., et al., Subepidermal vesicular dermatosis and sensory peripheral neuropathy caused by pyridoxine abuse, *J. Am. Acd. Dermatol.* 14:915-917, May 1986.

Gaby A., *The Doctor's Guide to Vitamin B6*, Rodale Press, Emmaus, Pennsylvania, 1984; Keats Publishing, New Canaan, Connecticut, 1987 (as *B6: The Natural Healer*).

Garber, C., et al., Immunomodulating properties of dimethylglycine in humans, *J. Inf. Dis.*, 143:101, 1981.

Garkin, I., et al., Pangamic acid and its derivatives, Inst. of Biochemistry, USSR Academy of Sciences, Moscow, 1964.

Gibbons G. F., et al., *Biochemistry of Cholesterol*, Elsevier Biomedical Press, New York, 1982.

Glick and Mayer, *Nature* (London), 218:1374, 1968.

Goldin, B. R., Gorbach, S. L., *American Journal of Clinical Nutrition*, 39:756-761, 1984.

Goodhart, R. S. and Shils, M. E., *Modern Nutrition in Health and Disease*, Lea & Febiger, Philadelphia, p. 477-478, 1973.

Gotto Jr., A. M., Some reflections on arteriosclerosis: past, present and future. *Circulation* 72:8-15, 1985.

Gruberg, E. R., and Raymond, S. A., *Beyond Cholesterol*, St. Martin's Press, New York, 1981.

Grusky, F. L., et al., The gastrointestinal absorption of unaltered protein in normal infants and in infants recovering from diarrhea, *Pediatrics*, 16:76?, 1955.

Hakami, N., et al., Neonatal megaloblastic anemia due to inherited transcobalamin 11 deficiency in two siblings, *New England Journal of Medicine*, vol. 285, no. 21:1163, 1971.

Harding, R. S. O., et al. (eds.), *Omnivorous Primates*, Columbia University Press, New York, 1981.

Harold, P. M., Kinsella, J. E., Fish oil consumption and decreased risk of cardiovascular disease: a comparison of findings from animal and human feeding trials, *Am. J. Clin. Nutr.*, 43:566-98, 1986.

Hetherington, A. W. and Ranson, S. W., Hypothalamic lesions and adiposity in the rat, *Anat. Rec.*, 78:149, 1940; and The spontaneous activity and food intake of rats with hypothalamic lesions, *Am. J. Physiol.*, 136:609, 1942.

Heinbecker, P., et al., Experimental obesity in the dog, *Am. J. Physiol.*, 141:549, 1944.

Heymann, C. D., *Poor Little Rich Girl: The Life and Legend of Barbara Hutton*, Pocket Books, New York, 1986.

Hendler, S. S., *The Complete Guide to Anti-Aging Nutrients*, Fireside Books, St. Louis, 1984.

Hicks, G. Richard, letter from Linus Pauling Institute of Science and Medicine, April 15, 1987.

Info World, Dec. 1, 1986.

Isaac, Glynn, The diet of early man, *World Archaeology*, Feb., 1971.

Jolly, C. J., and Plog, F., *Physical Anthropology and Archeology*, Alfred A. Knopf, New York, 1982.

Kirschbaum, W. R., Excessive hunger as a symptom of cerebral origin, *J. Nerv. & Ment. Dis.*, 113:95, 1951.

Krebs, E., et al., Pangamic sodium: a newly isolated crystalline water-soluble factor, *Int. Red. Med.*, 163:18, 1951.

Kromhout, D., Bosschieter, E. B., Coulander, C. D. The inverse relationship between fish consumption and 20-year mortality from heart disease. *New England J. Med.*, 312:1205-1209, 1985.

Kubo, T., *Arch. Exp. Zellforsch.*, 23:269, 1939.

Larrson, S., On the hypothalamic organization of the nervous mechanism regulating food intake. Part I: Hyperphagia from stimulation of the hypothalamus and medulla in sheep and goats, *Acta Physiol, Scandinav.*, 32:Suppl. 115, 1, 1954.

Levine, M., New concepts in the biology of biochemistry of ascorbic acid. *New England J. Med.*, 314:892-902, April 3, 1986.

Lieb, C. W., The effects on human beings of a twelve-month exclusive meat diet, *Journal of the American Medical Association*, July 9, 1929 and July 3, 1926, Stefansson examination report.

Lipid research clincs program: Lipid research clinics coronary primary prevention trial results. *Journal of the American Medical Association*, 251:351-374, 1984.

Lipkin, M., et al., The effect of added dietary calcium on colonic epithelial cell proliferation in subjects at high risk for familial colonic cancer, *New England J. Med.*, vol. 313, no. 22, Nov. 28, 1985.

Lippard, V. W., et al., Immune reactions induced in infants by intestinal absorption of incompletely digested cow's milk protein, *Am. J. Dis. Child.*, 51:562, 1936.

Lowering blood cholesterol to prevent heart disease: NIH Consensus Development Conference statement. *Arteriosclerosis*, 4:404-441, 1985.

London, R. S., et al., Hypothesis: breast cancer prevention by supplemental vitamin E, *Am. Coll. Nutr.*, 4:559-564, Sept.-Oct., 1985.

Marwich C., Campaign seeks to increase U.S. "cholesterol consciousness." *Journal of the American Medical Association*, 255:1097-1102, 1986.

Merck & Co., Rahway, N. J., Personal communication, 1985.

The Merck Manual, 14th Edition, Merck & Co., Inc., Rahway, 1982.

The Merck Manual, 13th Edition, Merck & Co., Inc., Rahway, 1977.

Milanino, R. et al., Review: copper and inflammation—a possible rationale for the pharmacological manipulation of inflammatory disorders. *Agents Actions*, 16:504-513, Sept. 1985 (Roberto Milanino, Institute of Pharmacology, University of Verona, Verona, Italy.).

Miller, D. R., and Hayes, K. C., Vitamin excess and toxicity, *Nutritional Toxicology*, Academic Press, Inc., New York, 1982.

Miller, N. E., Forde, O. H., Thelle, D. S., and Mijos, O. D., The Tromso Heart Study. High density lipoproteins and coronary heart disease: a prospective case-controlled study. *Lancet*, 1:965, 1977.

Mintz. S. W., *Sweetness and Power*, Viking, New York, 1985.

Morgane, P. K., Medical forebrain bundle and "feeding centers" of the hypothalamus, *J. Comp. Neurol.*, 117:1, 1961.

Nichols, A. B., et al., Independence of serum lipid levels and dietary habits, the Tecumseh study, *Journal of the American Medical Association*, 17:236, 1976.

Nizametidinova, G. A., Effectiveness of calcium pangamate introduced into vaccinated and X-irradiated animals. Reports of the Kazan Veterinary Institute, 112:100-104, 1972.

Packard, Jr., V. S., *Processed Foods and the Consumer*, University of Minnesota Press, Minneapolis, 1976.

Pauling, L., *Vitamin C and the Common Cold*, W. H. Freeman and Co., San Francisco, 1970.

Pinckney, E. R., The accuracy and significance of medical testing, *Archives of Internal Medicine*, March 1983.

Prange, Jr., A. J., Enhancement of imipramine antidepressant activity by thyroid hormone, *American Journal of Psychiatry*, vol. 126:4, Oct. 1969.

Randolph, T. G., Descriptive features of food addiction, addictive eating and drinking, *J. Stud. Alcohol*, 17:198, 1956.

Randolph, T. G., Masked food allergy as a factor in the development and persistence of obesity, *J. Lab. & Clin. Med.*, 32:1547, 1947.

Ratner, B. and Gruehl, H. L., Passage of native proteins through the gastrointestinal wall, *J. Clin. Invest.*, 13:517, 1934.

Rinkel, H. J., Randolph, T. G., and Zeller, M., *Food Allergy*, Charles C. Thomas, Springfield, 1951.

Reynolds, E. H., Neurological aspects of folate and vitamin B-12 metabolism, *Clin. Haematol.*, 5:661-696, 1976.

Rosenberg, L. E., Inherited defects of B-12 metabolism, *Science News of the Week*, 98:157-158, Aug. 22, 1970.

Rosenberg, L. E., Finding and treating genetic diseases, *Science News of the Week*, 98:157, Aug. 29, 1970.

Ross, F. C. and Campbell, A. H., The effects of vitamin A and vitamin D capsules upon the incidence of coronary heart disease and blood cholesterol, *Med. J. of Australia*, 48(2):307-311, Aug. 19, 1961.

Rowe, A. H., and Rose, A., *Food Allergy*, Charles C. Thomas, Springfield, 1972.

Royal Canadian Air Force Exercise Plan for Physical Fitness, Revised U.S. Edition. Pocket Books, New York, 1972.

Sanjo, K., *Folia Pharmacol.*, 17:219, Japan 1934.

Sanjo, K., Pharmacology, *Jap. J. Med. Sci. IV*, 9:13, 1936.

Sasaki, M., *Arch. Exp. Zellforsch.*, 21:289, 1938.

Schaumburg, H., et al., *The New England Journal of Medicine*, vol. 309, number 8:445, Aug. 25, 1983.

Schreurs, W. P. H., et al., The influence of radiotherapy and chemotherapy on the vitamin status of cancer patients, *Int. J. Nutr. Res.*, 55:425-432, Oct.-Dec., 1985.

Science News, vol. 127:268-69, April 27, 1985.

Semura, S., *Folia Pharmacol.*, 13:34, Japan 1933.

Sherman, H. C., et al., Vitamin A in relation to aging and to length of life, Proceedings of the National Academy of Science, vol. 31, no. 4:107-9, April 15, 1945.

Sherman, H. C., and Trupp, H. Y., Further experiments with vitamin A in relation to aging and length of life, Proceedings of the National Academy of Science, vol. 35:90-92, February 1949.

Sils, Ann, *N.Y. Acad. Sci.*, 162:847, 1969.

Smith, R. L., Pinckney, E. R., *Diet, Blood Cholesterol, And Coronary Heart Disease: A Critical Review of the Literature*, Victor Enterprises, Inc, Santa Monica, 1988.

Speer, F. (ed.), *Allergy of the Nervous System*, Charles C. Thomas, Springfield, 1970.

Stefansson, V., *Not By Bread Alone*, The Macmillan Company, New York, 1946.

Stone, I., *The Healing Factor*, Grossett & Dunlap, Inc., New York, 1972.

Teitelbaum, P. and Epstein, A. N., The lateral hypothalamic syndrome, recovery of feeding and drinking after lateral hypothalamic lesions, *Psychol. Rev.*, 69:74, 1962.

Thorn, W. H., et al. (eds.), *Harrison's Principles of Internal Medicine*, 8th Edition, McGraw-Hill, Inc., New York, 1977.

Toth, B., Synthetic and naturally occurring hydrazines as possible cancer causing agents, *Cancer Research*, p. 3693-97, Dec., 1975.

Van der Westhuyzen, J., Methionine metabolism and cancer, *Nutr. Cancer*, 7:179-183, July-Sept. 1985.

Wagner, D. A., et al., Effects of vitamins C and E on endogenous synthesis of N-nitrosamino acids in humans: precursor-product studies with [15N]nitrite, *Cancer Research*, 45:6519-6522, Dec. 1985.

Webster's Ninth New Collegiate Dictionary, Merriam-Webster Inc., Springfield, 1983.

West, J. B., *Best and Taylor's Physiological Basis of Medical Practice*, p. 839, 1227, 1235, Williams & Wilkins, Baltimore, 1985.

Wheatley, M. D., The hypothalamus and appetite behavior in cats: a study of the effects of experimental lesions with anatomical correlations, *Arch. Neurol. & Psychiat.*, 52:296, 1944.

Williams, R., *Nutrition Against Disease*, Pitman Publishing Co., New York, 1971.

Williams, R. J., *Biochemical Individuality: The Basis for the Genotrophic Concept*, Wiley, New York, 1956 (Univ. of Texas Press, Austin).

Witting, L. A., et al., The relationship of pyridoxine and riboflavin to the nutritional value of polymerized fats, *Journal of American Oil Chemists' Society*, p. 421-424, Sept., 1957.

World Health Organization, 1950, as quoted in Frederick G. Hoffman: *A Book on Drug and Alcohol Abuses, The Biochemical Aspects*, Oxford University Press, New York, 1975.

Yew, M. S., A plus for Pauling and vitamin C, *Science News*, May 5, 1973.

Index

One Final Word From the Author

Reading this book shows that you are serious about understanding the role of diet in your health. You might consider joining the Price-Pottenger Nutrition Foundation, which has been dispensing nutrition information since 1965. PPNF is dedicated to the proposition that the quality of our soil and the health and well-being of our plant and animal kingdoms determine the quality of human life.

The Foundation's name honors two internationally acclaimed nutrition researchers, Weston A. Price, D.D.S. and Francis M. Pottenger, Jr., M.D. Dr. Price's landmark work *Nutrition and Physical Degeneration* is, in my opinion, the second most important book ever written. If everyone read it and fully understood its implications, our world would be infinitely better.

For information, you may write or telephone

Price-Pottenger Nutrition Foundation
PO Box 2614
La Mesa, CA 91943-2614
(619) 582-4168